AIDS IN AFRICA:
A PANDEMIC ON THE MOVE

AIDS IN AFRICA:
A PANDEMIC ON THE MOVE

GARSON J. CLATON
EDITOR

Novinka Books
An imprint of Nova Science Publishers, Inc.
New York

Copyright © 2006 by Novinka Books
An imprint of Nova Science Publishers, Inc.

For permission to use material from this book please contact us:
Telephone 631-231-7269; Fax 631-231-8175
Web Site: http://www.novapublishers.com

NOTICE TO THE READER

The Publisher has taken reasonable care in the preparation of this book, but makes no expressed or implied warranty of any kind and assumes no responsibility for any errors or omissions. No liability is assumed for incidental or consequential damages in connection with or arising out of information contained in this book. The Publisher shall not be liable for any special, consequential, or exemplary damages resulting, in whole or in part, from the readers' use of, or reliance upon, this material.

This publication is designed to provide accurate and authoritative information with regard to the subject matter covered herein. It is sold with the clear understanding that the Publisher is not engaged in rendering legal or any other professional services. If legal or any other expert assistance is required, the services of a competent person should be sought. FROM A DECLARATION OF PARTICIPANTS JOINTLY ADOPTED BY A COMMITTEE OF THE AMERICAN BAR ASSOCIATION AND A COMMITTEE OF PUBLISHERS.

Library of Congress Cataloging-in-Publication Data:

Available Upon Request

ISBN: 1-59454-596-0

Published by Nova Science Publishers, Inc. ✤ *New York*

CONTENTS

PREFACE

Sub-Saharan Africa has been more severely affected by AIDS than any other part of the world. The United Nations reports that 25.4 million adults and children are infected with the HIV virus in the region, which has about 10% of the world's population but nearly 64% of the worldwide total of infected people. The overall rate of infection among adults in sub-Saharan Africa is 7.4%, compared with 1.1% worldwide. Ten countries in southern Africa have infection rates above 10% and account for 30% of infected adults worldwide. By the end of 2004, an estimated 25.3 million Africans will have died of AIDS, including a 2004 estimate of 2.3 million deaths. AIDS has surpassed malaria as the leading cause of death in Africa, and it kills many times more Africans than war. In Africa, 57% of those infected are women. Experts relate the severity of the African AIDS epidemic to the region's poverty, the relative lack of empowerment among women, high numbers of men living as migrant workers, and other factors. Health systems are ill-equipped for prevention, diagnosis, and treatment. AIDS' severe social and economic consequences are depriving Africa of skilled workers and teachers while reducing life expectancy by decades in some countries. An estimated 12.3 million AIDS orphans are currently living in Africa, facing increased risk of malnutrition and reduced prospects for education. AIDS is being blamed for declines in agricultural production in some countries, and is regarded as a major contributor to hunger and famine. Donor governments, non-governmental organizations, and African governments have responded through prevention programs intended to reduce the number of new infections and by trying to ameliorate the damage done by AIDS to families, societies, and economies. The adequacy of this response is the subject of much debate. An estimated 310,000 Africa AIDS patients were being treated with antiretroviral drugs at the end of 2004, up from 150,000 six months earlier. However, an estimated 4 million are in need of the therapy. U.S. and other initiatives are expected to sharply expand the availability of treatment in the near future. Advocates see expanded treatment as an affordable means of reducing the impact of the pandemic. Skeptics question whether treatment can be widely provided without costly improvements in health infrastructure. U.S. concern over AIDS in Africa grew during the 1980s, as the severity of the epidemic became apparent. Legislation enacted in the 106th and the 107th Congresses increased funding for worldwide HIV/AIDS programs. H.R. 1298, signed into law (P.L. 108-25) on May 27, 2003, authorized $15 billion over five years for international AIDS programs. President Bush announced his Emergency Plan for AIDS Relief (PEPFAR) in the 2003 State of the Union message. Twelve of the 15 focus countries are in sub-Saharan Africa. Under the FY2006 budget request, they would receive a 54% boost in aid, to $1.2 billion, through the State Department's Global HIV/AIDS Initiative. Nonetheless, activists and others urge that more be done in view of the scale of the African pandemic. This new book presents a nutshell analysis of this desperate situation.

In: Aids in Africa: A Pandemic on the Move   ISBN 1-59454-596-0
Editor: Garson J. Claton, pp. 1-24   © 2006 Nova Science Publishers, Inc.

Chapter 1

AIDS IN AFRICA

Raymond W. Copson

SUMMARY

Sub-Saharan Africa has been more severely affected by AIDS than any other part of the world. The United Nations reports that 25.4 million adults and children are infected with the HIV virus in the region, which has about 10% of the world's population but nearly 64% of the worldwide total of infected people. The overall rate of infection among adults in sub-Saharan Africa is 7.4%, compared with 1.1% worldwide. Ten countries in southern Africa have infection rates above 10% and account for 30% of infected adults worldwide. By the end of 2004, an estimated 25.3 million Africans will have died of AIDS, including a 2004 estimate of 2.3 million deaths. AIDS has surpassed malaria as the leading cause of death in Africa, and it kills many times more Africans than war. In Africa, 57% of those infected are women.

Experts relate the severity of the African AIDS epidemic to the region's poverty, the relative lack of empowerment among women, high numbers of men living as migrant workers, and other factors. Health systems are ill-equipped for prevention, diagnosis, and treatment.

AIDS' severe social and economic consequences are depriving Africa of skilled workers and teachers while reducing life expectancy by decades in some countries. An estimated 12.3 million AIDS orphans are currently living in Africa, facing increased risk of malnutrition and reduced prospects for education. AIDS is being blamed for declines in agricultural production in some countries, and is regarded as a major contributor to hunger and famine.

Donor governments, non-governmental organizations, and African governments have responded through prevention programs intended to reduce the number of new infections and by trying to ameliorate the damage done by AIDS to families, societies, and economies. The adequacy of this response is the subject of much debate.

An estimated 310,000 Africa AIDS patients were being treated with antiretroviral drugs at the end of 2004, up from 150,000 six months earlier. However, an estimated 4 million are in need of the therapy. U.S. and other initiatives are expected to sharply expand the availability of treatment in the near future. Advocates see expanded treatment as an affordable means of reducing the impact of the pandemic. Skeptics question whether treatment can be widely provided without costly improvements in health infrastructure.

U.S. concern over AIDS in Africa grew during the 1980s, as the severity of the epidemic became apparent. Legislation enacted in the 106th and the 107th Congresses increased funding for worldwide HIV/AIDS programs. H.R. 1298, signed into law (P.L. 108-25) on May 27, 2003, authorized $15 billion over five years for international AIDS programs. President Bush announced his Emergency Plan for AIDS Relief (PEPFAR) in the 2003 State of the Union message. Twelve of the 15 focus countries are in sub-Saharan Africa. Under the FY2006 budget request, they would receive a 54% boost in aid, to $1.2 billion, through the State Department's Global HIV/AIDS Initiative. Nonetheless, activists and others urge that more be done in view of the scale of the African pandemic.

MOST RECENT DEVELOPMENTS

Senator Frist introduced S. 850 on April 19, 2005, to authorize a Global Health Corps that would send U.S. health volunteers abroad and expand the availability of health care personnel, items, and related services. That same day, the National Academies' Institute of Medicine (IOM) released a report calling for a United States Global Health Service to mobilize health personnel to work in the 15 focus countries of the President's Emergency Plan for AIDS Relief (PEPFAR) in order to help achieve PEPFAR's goals. An initial deployment of 150 key professionals would be paid full salary; others would receive $35,000 fellowships and student loan repayments up to $25,000. Some suggested that funds might better be spent training and retaining indigenous health personnel, particularly in Africa; others noted that training was a key component of the IOM proposal, which they praised as a dynamic response to the AIDS crisis. The House Committee on International Relations held a hearing on April 13 on the U.S. response to the global AIDS crisis. Chairman Henry Hyde praised U.S. AIDS Coordinator Randall Tobias for "tremendous leadership" but called for more support for organizations devoted to promoting abstinence and being faithful. On April 11, former President Bill Clinton announced that the Clinton Foundation was launching a pediatric AIDS program that would put 10,000 children on antiretroviral AIDS therapy in at least 10 countries in 2005 — doubling the number of children in treatment.

BACKGROUND AND ANALYSIS

Sub-Saharan Africa has been far more severely affected by AIDS than any other part of the world. In December 2004, UNAIDS (the Joint United Nations Program on HIV/AIDS) reported that in 2004, 25.4 million adults and children were living with HIV and AIDS in the region, including 3.1 million newly infected during the year. Africa has about 10% of the world's population but approximately 64% of the worldwide total of infected people. The infection rate among adults aged 15-49 averages an estimated 7.4% in Africa, compared with 1.1% worldwide. According to cumulative UNAIDS estimates, approximately 25.3 million Africans will have died of AIDS since the beginning of the epidemic through the end of 2004, including an estimated 2.3 million expected to die in that year. UNAIDS projects that between 2000 and 2020, 55 million Africans can be expected to lose their lives to the epidemic. (*Report on the Global HIV/AIDS Epidemic, 2002*, p. 46.) AIDS has surpassed malaria as the leading cause of death in sub-Saharan Africa, and it kills many times more people than Africa's armed conflicts.

CHARACTERISTICS OF THE AFRICAN EPIDEMIC

- HIV, the human immunodeficiency virus that causes AIDS, is spread in Africa primarily by heterosexual contact. (A February 2003 article published by David Gisselquist and others in the *International Journal of STD and AIDS* asserted that the importance of unsafe medical practices in the spread of HIV may have been underestimated. A February 2004 article in *The Lancet* rejected this hypothesis, and affirmed that sexual transmission "continues to be the major mode of spread" of HIV.[1])

- Women make up an estimated 57% of the HIV-positive adult population in sub-Saharan Africa, as compared with 47% worldwide, according to UNAIDS. Young women are particularly at risk. In 2004, an estimated 6.9% of African women aged 15 to 24 were HIV positive, compared with 2.2% of young men. (UNAIDS, *AIDS Epidemic Update, December 2004).*

- According to UNAIDS, the adult infection rate or prevalence has stabilized in sub-Saharan Africa in recent years, as both the total adult population and the number of infected people increase. Stabilization does not ease the burden of the epidemic but simply means that numbers dying approximately equal the numbers of newly infected. The disease has become endemic in many countries and will affect their people for generations to come. Prevalence is still increasing in Madagascar, Swaziland, and a few other countries, while Uganda and localized areas in some other countries have experienced declines.

- Southern Africa, where 10 countries have an adult infection rate above 10% (**Table 1**), is the most severely affected region. With 2% of the world's population, these countries account for nearly 30% of infected people worldwide. However, populous Nigeria in West Africa, where an estimated 5.4% of adults are infected, has an estimated 3.6 million infected people —the largest number in the region apart from South Africa, where UNAIDS estimates that 5.3 million are infected. South Africa's is the largest infected population in the world.

- The African AIDS epidemic is having a much greater impact on children than is the case in other parts of the world. According to UNAIDS, more than 600,000 African infants become infected with HIV each year through mother-to-child transmission, either at birth or through breast-feeding. Most die before their second birthday. Nonetheless, an estimated 1.9 million African children under 14 were living with AIDS at the end of 2003. In South Africa, a sample survey reported by the Human Sciences Research Council in May 2004 showed that 6.7% of children between the ages of 2 and 9 were HIV positive.

- In 2003, there were an estimated 12.3 million AIDS orphans in Africa —that is, children 17 and under who had lost one or both parents to the disease.[2] Because of the stigma attached to the AIDS disease, AIDS orphans are at high risk for being malnourished, abused, and denied an education. In November 2003, UNICEF released a report, *Africa's Orphaned Generations*, predicting that there would be 20 million AIDS orphans in Africa by 2010 and that in a dozen countries orphans from all causes would account for 15% to more than 25% of children under 15. Among other measures, the report recommended efforts to strengthen the capacity of families to protect and care for orphans.

Table 1. Adult HIV Infection Rates (%), end of 2003

Swaziland	38.8	Tanzania	8.8	Chad	4.8	Eritrea	2.7
Botswana	37.3	Gabon	8.1	Ethiopia	4.4	Sudan	2.3
Lesotho	28.9	Cote d'Ivoire	7.0	Burkina Faso	4.2	Mali	1.9
Zimbabwe	24.6	Cameroon	6.9	Congo Kinshasa	4.2	Benin	1.9
South Africa	21.5	Kenya	6.7	Uganda	4.1	Madagascar	1.7
Namibia	21.3	Burundi	6.0	Togo	4.1	Gambia	1.2
Zambia	16.5	Liberia	5.9	Angola	3.9	Niger	1.2
Malawi	14.2	Nigeria	5.4	Guinea	3.2	Senegal	.8
Central Af. Rep.	13.5	Rwanda	5.1	Ghana	3.1		
Mozambique	12.2	Congo Brazzaville	4.9	Djibouti	2.9		

Source: UNAIDS, Report on the Global HIV/AIDS Epidemic, July 2002. The Zimbabwe estimate represents a technical correction issued in 2003. Updated estimates are expected in July 2004.

EXPLAINING THE AFRICAN EPIDEMIC

AIDS experts emphasize a variety of economic and social factors in explaining Africa's AIDS epidemic, placing primary blame on the region's poverty. Poverty has deprived Africa of effective systems of health information, health education, and health care. Thus, Africans suffer from a high rate of untreated sexually-transmitted infections (STIs) other than AIDS, and these increase susceptibility to HIV. African health systems typically have limited capabilities for AIDS prevention work, and HIV counseling and testing are difficult for many Africans to obtain. Until very recently, AIDS treatment has been generally available only to the elite.

Poverty forces large numbers of African men to migrate long distances in search of work, and while away from home they may have multiple sex partners, increasing their risk of infection. Some of these partners may be women who have become commercial sex workers because of poverty, and they too are highly vulnerable to infection. Migrant workers may carry the infection back to their wives when they return home. Long distance truck drivers, and drivers of "taxis," who transport Africans long distances by car, are probably also key agents in spreading HIV. Meanwhile, poverty forces many women to turn to "transactional sex" in order to survive.

Some behavior patterns in Africa may also be affecting the epidemic. In explaining the fact that young women are infected at a higher rate than young men, Peter Piot, the Executive Director UNAIDS, has commented that "the unavoidable conclusion is that girls are getting infected not by boys but by older men," who are more likely than young men to carry the disease. (UNAIDS press release, September 14, 1999.) UNAIDS notes that "with the downward trend of many African economies ... relationships with (older) men can serve as vital opportunities for financial and social security, or for satisfying material aspirations." (*AIDS Epidemic Update, 2002).* Many believe that the infection rate among women generally would be far lower if women's rights were more widely respected in Africa, if women exercised more power in political and economic affairs, and if donors and governments would support fidelity campaigns primarily aimed at African men. (For more on these issues, see Helen Epstein, "AIDS: the Lesson of Uganda," *New York Review of Books*, July 5, 2001; "The Hidden Cause of AIDS," *New York Review of Books*, May 9, 2002; and "The Fidelity Fix," *New York Times Magazine*, June 13, 2004.) A Human Rights Watch study released on August 13, 2003, reported that domestic violence made women in Uganda more vulnerable to HIV infection — for example by depriving them of the power to negotiate condom use.

LEADERSHIP REACTION IN
SOUTH AFRICA AND ELSEWHERE

Many observers believe that the spread of AIDS in Africa could have been slowed if African leaders had been more engaged and outspoken in earlier stages of the epidemic. President Thabo Mbeki of South Africa has come in for particular criticism on this score. In April 2000, President Mbeki wrote then President Clinton and other heads of state defending dissident scientists who maintain that AIDS is not caused by the HIV virus. In March 2001, Mbeki rejected appeals that the national assembly declare the AIDS pandemic a national emergency.

Under mounting domestic and international pressure, the South African government seemed to modify its position significantly when the government announced after an April 2002 cabinet meeting that it would triple the national AIDS budget. When a treatment program had not been launched by March 2003, however, the Treatment Action Campaign (TAC) launched a civil disobedience campaign. In August 2003, the South African cabinet instructed the health ministry to develop a plan to provide antiretroviral therapy nationwide, but by March 2004, TAC was threatening a lawsuit unless the program was actually begun. Finally, on April 1, 2004, the government began offering treatment at 5 hospitals in Gauteng province, centered on Johannesburg. TAC reported in February 2005 that about 70,000 South Africans were receiving treatment, but of these only 27,000 were being treated through the public program, while the remainder were under private care. An estimated 500,000 South Africans are in need of treatment.

The delays in South Africa's response to the pandemic have been costly, many experts believe. On September 22, 2004, South Africa's Department of Health reported survey results indicating that HIV infection was continuing to spread, though at a somewhat slower rate than in previous years. Approximately 27.9% of pregnant women in South Africa were found to be HIV positive in 2003, up from 26.5% in 2002. The department estimated that 5.6 million South Africans were infected. A report released by the Bureau of Market Research at the University of South Africa on September 20, 2004, predicted that AIDS-related deaths would exceed 500,000 per year from 2007 through 2011. Nonetheless, South Africa's Health Minister Manto Tshabalala Msimang continues to question the effectiveness of antiretrovirals and to insist that a healthy diet, particularly one including raw garlic and lemon peel, can offer protection from the disease. (*Mail and Guardian Online*, May 5, 2005). Former President Nelson Mandela, seeking to combat the stigma and secrecy associated with AIDS, announced on January 6, 2005, that his son, Makgatho, had died of the disease.

In the rest of Africa, many heads of state and other leaders are now taking major roles in fighting the epidemic. President Yoweri Museveni of Uganda has long been recognized for leading a successful prevention campaign against AIDS in his country, and Uganda's ABC (Abstinence, Be Faithful, or Use Condoms) transmission prevention program has won wide praise. ("Uganda Leads by Example on AIDS," *Washington Times*, March 13, 2003.) A Senate Foreign Relations Africa Subcommittee hearing on May 19, 2003, focused on "Fighting AIDS in Uganda: What Went Right." Dr. Anne Peterson, Assistant Administrator for Global Health at the U.S. Agency for International Development (USAID), testified that the "Uganda success story is about prevention." She said that successes had been recorded in promoting abstinence and faithfulness to partners, while increased condom use in recent years had also contributed to the decline in prevalence. Sophia Mukasa Monico, a member of the Global Health Council and a former AIDS worker in Uganda, testified that all three program elements need to be in place for prevention to work. Mukasa Monico noted that "the epidemic is still raging in Uganda, and we have much to do before we can claim victory...." On February 23, 2005, researchers from Johns Hopkins and Columbia University released a study from Rakai, Uganda, finding that a decline in HIV prevalence there was due to condom use and the deaths of infected people.[3] Abstinence and monogamy appeared not to be increasing. Some saw this as evidence that programs to encourage sexual behavior change were less important than expected, while others argued that behavior had likely already changed substantially before the study began.

The presidents of Botswana, Nigeria, and several other countries are widely seen today as in the forefront of the AIDS struggle as well. Several regional AIDS initiatives have been launched. For example, in August 2003, the Southern African Development Community (SADC) agreed to an AIDS strategic framework, including the creation of a regional fund to fight the disease.

SOCIAL AND ECONOMIC CONSEQUENCES

AIDS is having severe social and economic consequences in Africa, and these negative effects are expected to continue for many years. A January 2000 Central Intelligence Agency National Intelligence Estimate on the infectious disease threat, made public in an unclassified version, forecasts grave problems over the next 20 years.

> At least some of the hardest-hit countries, initially in sub-Saharan Africa and later in other regions, will face a demographic catastrophe as HIV/AIDS and associated diseases reduce human life expectancy dramatically and kill up to a quarter of their populations over the period of this Estimate. This will further impoverish the poor, and often the middle class, and produce a huge and impoverished orphan cohort unable to cope and vulnerable to exploitation and radicalization. (CIA, *The Global Infectious Disease Threat and Its Implications for the United States* [http://www.odci.gov], "Publications and Reports".)

The estimate predicted increased political instability and slower democratic development as a result of AIDS. According to the World Bank,

The illness and impending death of up to 25% of all adults in some countries will have an enormous impact on national productivity and earnings. Labor productivity is likely to drop, the benefits of education will be lost, and resources that would have been used for investments will be used for health care, orphan care, and funerals. Savings rates will decline, and the loss of human capital will affect production and the quality of life for years to come. (World Bank, *Intensifying Action Against HIV/AIDS in Africa.*)

In the most severely affected countries, sharp drops in life expectancy are occurring, and these will reverse major gains achieved in recent decades. According to UNAIDS, as a result of AIDS, average life expectancy in sub-Saharan Africa is now 47 years, whereas it would have been 62 years without the epidemic. A U.S. Bureau of the Census report [http://www.census.gov/prod/2004pubs/wp02-2.pdf], released on March 23, 2004, predicted population declines by 2010 in South Africa, Botswana, and three other African countries due to AIDS.

According to many reports, AIDS has devastating effects on rural families. The father is typically the first to fall ill, and when this occurs, farm tools and animals may be sold to pay for his care. Should the mother also become ill, children may be forced to shoulder responsibility for the full time care of their parents. The Food and Agriculture Organization of the United Nations reports that since the epidemic began, 7 million agricultural workers have been killed in Africa. The agricultural workforce has been reduced by more than 20% in five countries (FAO, *HIV/AIDS, Food Security, and Rural Livelihoods*, May 2002), and a number of experts are relating serious food shortages in southern Africa in 2002 and 2003 to production losses caused by AIDS. (See "Cursed Twice Over — AIDS and Famine in Southern Africa," *The Economist*, February 15, 2003.) World Food Program Executive Director James Morris, testifying before the Senate Foreign Relations Committee on February 25, 2003, and the House International Relations Committee on February 27, said that HIV/AIDS was a central cause of the famine. On June 22, 2004, Morris said that southern Africa was in a "death spiral" due to the consequences of the AIDS pandemic, including the loss of human capacity and the devastation of rural areas, with resulting negative consequences for food security (WFP press release).

AIDS is being blamed for shortages of skilled workers and teachers in several countries. A May 2002 World Bank study, *Education and HIV/AIDS: A Window of Hope,* reported that more than 30% of teachers are HIV positive in parts of Malawi and Uganda, 20% in Zambia, and 12% in South Africa. AIDS is also claiming many lives at middle and upper levels of management in both business and government. Although unemployment is generally high in Africa, trained personnel are not readily replaced.

AIDS may have serious security consequences for much of Africa, since HIV infection rates in many armies are extremely high. Domestic political stability could also be threatened in African countries if the security forces become unable to perform their duties due to AIDS. Peacekeeping is also at risk. South African soldiers are expected to play an important peacekeeping role in Africa in the years ahead, but this could be threatened. Estimates of the infection rate in the South Africa army run from 17% to 40%, with higher rates reported for units based in heavily infected KwaZulu-Natal province.

RESPONSES TO THE AIDS EPIDEMIC

Donor governments, non-governmental organizations (NGOs) working in Africa, and African governments have responded to the AIDS epidemic primarily by attempting to reduce the number of new HIV infections through prevention programs, and to some degree, by trying to ameliorate the damage done by AIDS to families, societies, and economies. A third response, treatment of AIDS sufferers with antiretroviral drugs that can result in long-term survival, has not been widely used in Africa until recently; but treatment programs are expanding. (See below, **AIDS Treatment Issues**).

Programs and projects aimed at combating the epidemic typically provide information on how HIV is spread and on how it can be avoided through the media, posters, lectures, and skits. Some success has been claimed for these efforts in persuading young people to delay the age of "sexual debut" and to remain faithful to a single partner. The United States is now advocating an expansion of prevention programs focusing on abstinence until marriage as an effective means of slowing the spread of HIV, although some critics maintain that this may be unrealistic in a social environment destabilized by poverty. Some also question whether approaches stressing abstinence and faithfulness can benefit poor married women in Africa, who have little power to deny their husbands, whether infected or not.

Donor-sponsored voluntary counseling and testing (VCT) programs, where available, enable African men and women to learn their HIV status. In Botswana, HIV tests are now offered as a routine part of any medical visit, and many experts are urging that this be done continent-wide. AIDS awareness programs can be found in many African schools and increasingly in the workplace, where employers are recognizing their interest in reducing the infection rate among their employees. Many projects aim at making condoms readily available and on providing instruction in condom use. Several projects have had success in reducing mother-to-child transmission by administering the anti-HIV drug AZT or nevirapine, before and during birth, and while the mother is nursing. Many AIDS activists argue that it would be far better to put all infected pregnant women into long-term treatment programs, which would reduce the likelihood that their children would be orphaned.

On December 13, 2004, the Associated Press (AP) reported that a number of flaws had been found in a study of the nevirapine conducted in Uganda under the sponsorship of the National Institutes of Health (NIH). According to the AP report, researchers acknowledged that thousands of bad reactions were not disclosed. The allegations provoked criticism in Africa, including a furious response from the South Africa's ruling Africa National Congress (ANC). In a December 17 statement, the ANC charged that top U.S. officials had "entered into a conspiracy with a pharmaceutical company to tell lies and promote the sales of nevirapine in Africa ..." That same day, NIH issued its own statement affirming that "single-dose nevirapine is a safe and effective drug for preventing mother to infant transmission of HIV." The statement termed as "absolutely false" any implication of thousands of adverse reactions in the Uganda study. AIDS activists and others were concerned that the controversy would discourage use of the drug, often the only available means of preventing mother to child transmission (MTCT) of HIV. The National Academies' Institute of Medicine, after investigating the Uganda study, reported that the Uganda study was valid and that nevirapine should continue to be used for MTCT.

Church groups and humanitarian organizations have helped Africa deal with the consequences of AIDS by setting up programs to provide care and education to orphans. Public-private partnerships have also become an important vehicle for responding to the African AIDS pandemic. The Bill and Melinda Gates Foundation has been a major supporter of vaccine research and a variety of AIDS programs undertaken in cooperation with African governments and donors. The Rockefeller Foundation, working with UNAIDS and others, has sponsored programs to improve AIDS care in Africa, and both Bristol-Myers Squibb and Merck and Company, together with the Gates Foundation and the Harvard AIDS Institute, have undertaken programs with the Botswana government aimed at improving the country's health infrastructure and providing AIDS treatment to all who need it. In Uganda, Pfizer and the Pfizer Foundation are funding the Infectious Diseases

Institute (IDI), expected to train 250 AIDS treatment specialists annually, many of whom will work in rural areas.

The Global Fund to Fight AIDS, Tuberculosis, and Malaria, created in January 2002, commits about 60% of its grant funds to Africa, and about 60% of its grants worldwide go toward fighting AIDS. For further information, see CRS Report RL31712, *The Global Fund to Fight AIDS, Tuberculosis, and Malaria: Background and Current Issues*.

Nonetheless, UNAIDS maintains that a significant funding gap remains. In September 2003, the organization issued a report entitled *Accelerating Action Against AIDS in Africa*, which estimated that $8 billion was required to fight the African AIDS epidemic in 2004, whereas $6 billion was likely to be provided from all sources, including donors, the Global Fund, African governments, and African households. UNAIDS expects the resource gap to widen further in 2005. In January 2005, Gordon Brown, Britain's Chancellor of the Exchequer, proposed a $10 billion per year program to revitalize the struggle against AIDS. Many AIDS activists welcomed the proposal, but some said it would focus too heavily on vaccine research, which they regard as problematic.

Further information on the response to AIDS in Africa may be found below under **AIDS Treatment Issues** and at the following websites:

- CDC: [http://www.cdc.gov/nchstp/od/nchstp.html]
- Global Fund to Fight AIDS, Tuberculosis, and Malaria: [http://www.theglobalfund.org/en/]
- International AIDS Vaccine Initiative: [http://www.iavi.org] International Association of Physicians in AIDS Care: [http://www.iapac.org/]
- Kaiser Daily HIV/AIDS Report: [http://www.kaisernetwork.org/daily_reports/rep_hiv.cfm/]
- UNAIDs: [http://www.unaids.org/en/default.asp]
- USAID: [http://www.usaid.gov/], click on "Health." World Bank: [http://www.worldbank.org/], click on "Topics."

Effectiveness of the Response

The response to AIDS in Africa has had some successes, most notably in Uganda, where the rate of infection among pregnant women in urban areas fell from 29.5% in 1992 to 5% in 2001 (UNAIDS, *AIDS Epidemic Update, December 2002*). The infection rate has continued to drop, and in

2003, adult prevalence nationwide was 4.1%, compared with 5.1% in 2001. HIV prevalence among young urban women in Zambia has also reportedly fallen, and UNAIDS indicates that urban sexual behavior patterns among young people in cities in other countries may be changing in ways that combat the spread of HIV. (However, increases in infection rates continue in cities in several other countries.) South Africa has recorded a drop in infections among pregnant women under 20, and Senegal is credited with preventing an AIDS epidemic through an active, government-sponsored prevention program. Despite some success stories, however, the number of infected people in Africa continues to grow.

Experts point out that there are a number of barriers to a more effective AIDS response in Africa, such as cultural norms that make it difficult for many government, religious, and community leaders to acknowledge or discuss sexual matters, including sex practices, prostitution, and the use of condoms. However, experts continue to advocate AIDS awareness and AIDS amelioration as essential components of the response to the epidemic. Indeed, there is strong support for an intensification of awareness and amelioration efforts, as well as adaptations to make such efforts more effective.

The lives of infected people could be significantly prolonged and improved, some maintain, if more were done to identify and treat the opportunistic infections, particularly tuberculosis, that typically accompany AIDS. Millions of Africans suffer dual infections of HIV and TB, and the combined infection dramatically shortens life. Tuberculosis can be cured by treatment with a combination of medications over several months, even in HIV-infected patients. However, according to the World Health Organization, Africans often delay seeking treatment for TB or do not complete the course of medication (*Global Tuberculosis Control: WHO Report 1999,* Key Findings), contributing to the high incidence of death among those with dual infections. Pfizer Corporation has signed an agreement with South Africa to donate the anti-fungal Diflucan (fluconazole) for treating AIDS-related opportunistic infections, including cryptococcal meningitis, a dangerous brain inflammation. On December 1, 2001, Pfizer announced that it would sign memoranda of understanding on donating fluconazole with six other African countries. UNAIDS and the World Health organization have recommended that Africans infected with HIV be treated with an antibiotic/sulfa drug combination known by the trade name Bactrim in order to prevent opportunistic infections. Studies indicate that the drug could reduce AIDS death rates at a cost of between $8 and $17 per year per patient.

AIDS Treatment Issues

Access for poor Africans to antiretrovirals (ARVs) has been perhaps the most contentious issue surrounding the response to the African epidemic today. Administered in a treatment regimen known as HAART (highly active antiretroviral therapy) these drugs can return AIDS victims to normal life and permit long-term survival rather than early death. Such treatment has proven highly effective in developed countries, including the United States, where AIDS, which had been the eighth leading cause of death in 1996, no longer ranked among the 15 leading causes by 1998. (U.S. Department of Health and Human Services Press Release, October 5, 1999.)

The high cost of HAART treatments has been the principal obstacle to offering the therapy on a large scale in Africa, where most victims are poor and lack health insurance. The cost of administering HAART was once estimated at between $10,000 and $15,000 per person per year. In May 2000, five major pharmaceutical companies announced that they were willing to negotiate sharp reductions in the price of AIDS drugs sold in Africa. UNAIDS launched a program in cooperation with the pharmaceutical companies to boost treatment access and, in June 2001, reported that 10 African countries had reached agreement with manufacturers. The agreements significantly reduced prices in exchange for health infrastructure improvements to assure that ARVs are administered safely.

Initiatives to expand the availability of HAART continued, and treatment became a major focus of the programs of the Global Fund and of the President's Emergency Plan for AIDS Relief (PEPFAR, see below). On December 1, 2003, the World Health Organization formally launched its $5.5 billion "3 by 5" plan to treat 3 million AIDS patients in poor countries by 2005, with resources to come from the Global Fund and donors. Earlier, in October 2003, former President Bill Clinton announced that his foundation had organized a program to provide generic three-drug antiretroviral treatment for AIDS patients in Africa and the Caribbean for about $.38 per day. Generic pharmaceutical manufacturers in India and South Africa would make the drugs, and funding would come from private donors, some donor governments, and other sources. In April 2004, the Clinton Foundation announced an agreement with UNICEF, the World Bank, and the Global Fund to expand the program to more than 100 developing countries worldwide. As a result of the impending increased availability of treatment, an estimated 310,000 sub-Saharan patients were receiving HAART at the end of 2004, up from 150,000 six months earlier.[4] However, an estimated 4 million Africans are in need of HAART.

Dr. Jim Yong Kim, director of HIV/AIDS programs at WHO, said in February 2005 that the 3 by 5 campaign was struggling to attain its goal.[5] In Africa, Botswana and Uganda would likely meet their targets, but South Africa and Nigeria were lagging behind. South African Health Minister Tshabalala-Msimang said on May 5 that some were trying to "scapegoat" South Africa for the failure of 3 by 5 and that South Africa could not do a blanket rollout of antiretrovirals because patients had to be closely monitored due to side effects. She added that she would continue to inform patients that they had three options: improving nutrition, taking micronutrients, or enrolling in an antiretroviral program. (*Mail and Guardian Online*, May 5, 2005.)

Whether African countries are ready to "absorb" dramatically increased funding for treatment has been another issue. AIDS activists believe that millions of Africans could quickly be given access to AIDS drugs. Others maintain that African supply channels cannot make the drugs consistently available to millions of patients and that regular monitoring of patients by medical personnel is not possible in much of the continent. Monitoring is necessary, they maintain, to deal with side effects and to adjust medications if drug resistance emerges. Many fear that if the drugs are taken irregularly, resistant HIV strains will emerge that could cause untreatable infections worldwide; although a September 2003 report indicated that African patients follow their AIDS therapy regimens more consistently than American patients.[6] For some, the correct response to weaknesses in Africa's basic health care systems is to devote resources to strengthening those systems.[7]

Botswana's President Mogae told a November 12, 2003 meeting, convened in Washington by the Center for Strategic and International Studies, that the widely-praised treatment program in his country is being hampered by a "brain drain" of health personnel. Physicians, nurses, technicians, and other are often hired away by foreign governments, international organizations, and non-governmental organizations. The health minister of Mozambique, which has launched a pilot antiretroviral treatment program, said in May 2004 that the country was unable to launch a nationwide program because of serious shortages of staff and equipment. The Harvard-based Joint Learning Initiative on Human Resources for Health and Development issued a report on November 27, 2004 finding that Africa had the lowest ratio of health workers to population of any region. At least one million new workers are needed, according to the report. On December 3, 2004, Britain announced that it would provide $100 million to boost salaries of health workers in Malawi and increase the number of medical staff being trained.

AIDS activists have urged that African governments issue "compulsory licenses" to allow the manufacture or importation of inexpensive generic copies of patented AIDS medications. In November 2001, a ministerial-level meeting of the World Trade Organization(WTO) in Doha, Qatar, approved a declaration stating that the Agreement on Trade-Related Aspects of Intellectual Property Rights (TRIPS agreement) should be implemented in a manner supportive of promoting access to medicines for all. The declaration affirmed the right of countries to issue compulsory licenses and gave the least developed countries until 2016 to implement TRIPS. The question of whether countries manufacturing generic copies of patented drugs, such as India or Thailand, should be permitted to export to poor countries was left for further negotiation through a committee known as the Council for TRIPS.

Although the Doha declaration drew broad praise, some AIDS activists criticized it for not permitting imports of generics. Some in the pharmaceutical industry, on the other hand, expressed concern that the declaration was too permissive and might reduce profits that, they argued, were used to fund research. Others, however, maintained that the declaration would have little practical impact, because in their view, poverty rather than patents is the principal obstacle to drug access in Africa. (See Amir Attaran and Lee Gillespie-White, "Do Patents for Anti-retroviral Drugs Constrain Access to AIDS Treatment in Africa?" *Journal of the American Medical Association*, October 17, 2001.) On August 30, 2003, the WTO reached agreement on a plan to allow poor countries to import generic copies of essential medications, but the debate over access to antiretrovirals in Africa seems likely to continue. In March 2005, India's parliament completed passage of patent legislation expected to sharply raise prices in Africa and elsewhere for Indian-manufactured generic copies of newly discovered AIDS medications. Cheap generic copies of existing medications can still be sold, although sellers will have to pay licensing fees to patent holders.

U.S. POLICY

U.S. concern over AIDS in Africa began to mount during the 1980s, as the severity of the epidemic became apparent. In 1987, in acting on the FY1988 foreign operations appropriations, Congress earmarked funds for fighting AIDS worldwide, and House appropriators noted that in Africa, AIDS had the potential for "undermining all development efforts" to date (H.Rept. 100-283). In subsequent years, Congress supported AIDS spending at or above levels requested by the executive branch, either through earmarks or report language. Nevertheless, a widely discussed July 2000 *Washington Post* article called into question the adequacy and timeliness of the early U.S. response to the HIV/AIDS threat in Africa. (Barton Gellman, "The Global Response to AIDS in Africa: World Shunned Signs of Coming Plague." *Washington Post,* July 5, 2000. See also Greg Behrman, *The Invisible People: How the U.S. Has Slept Through the Global AIDS Pandemic, the Greatest Humanitarian Catastrophe of Our Time* (New York: Free Press, 2004).

As the severity of the epidemic continued to deepen, many of those concerned for Africa's future, both inside and outside government, came to feel that more should be done. On July 19, 1999, then Vice President Al Gore proposed $100 million in additional spending for a global LIFE (Leadership and Investment in Fighting an Epidemic) AIDS initiative to begin in FY2000, with a heavy focus on Africa. Funds approved during the FY2000 appropriations process supported most of this initiative. On June 27, 2000, the Peace Corps announced that all volunteers serving in Africa would be trained as AIDS educators.

USAID reported in 2001 that it had been the global leader in the international response to AIDS since 1986, not only by supporting multilateral efforts but also by directly sponsoring regional and bilateral programs aimed at combating the disease. (USAID,

Leading the Way: USAID Responds to HIV/AIDS, September 2001). The Agency had sponsored AIDS education programs; trained AIDS educators, counselors, and clinicians; supported condom distribution; and sponsored AIDS research. USAID claimed several successes in Africa, such as helping to reduce HIV prevalence among young Ugandans and to prevent an outbreak of the epidemic in Senegal; reducing the frequency of sexually transmitted infections in several African countries; sharply increasing condom availability in Kenya and elsewhere; assisting children orphaned by AIDS; and sponsoring the development of useful new technologies, including the female condom. USAID reported that it spent a total of $51 million on fighting AIDS in Africa in FY1998 and $63 million in FY1999 (*Leading the Way*, 121). In addition, some spending by the Department of Health and Human Services was going toward HIV surveillance in Africa and other Africa AIDS-related efforts.

Bush Administration

Combating the AIDS pandemic in sub-Saharan Africa has been an important focus for the Bush Administration's foreign assistance program. In May 2001, President Bush made the "founding pledge" of $200 million to the Global Fund, and on June 19, 2002, he announced a $500 million International Mother and Child HIV Prevention Initiative (IMCPI) to support programs to prevent mother-to-child transmission of the virus. Eight African countries were named as beneficiaries.

The President's Emergency Plan for AIDS Relief (PEPFAR) is resulting in major spending increases for HIV/AIDS prevention, care, and treatment in 12 focus countries in Africa: Botswana, Cote d'Ivoire, Ethiopia, Kenya, Mozambique, Namibia, Nigeria, Rwanda, South Africa, Tanzania, Uganda, and Zambia. (The other focus countries are Guyana, Haiti, and Vietnam.) President Bush announced the launching of PEPFAR in his January 2003 State of the Union address, pledging $15 billion for fiscal years 2004 through 2008, including $10 billion in "new money," that is, spending in addition to then current levels. The program aims to prevent 7 million new infections worldwide, provide anti-retroviral drugs for 2 million infected people, and provide care for 10 million infected people, including orphans. The new funds are coming through the Global HIV/AIDS Initiative (GHAI), headquartered at the Department of State. The GHAI is headed by the United States Global AIDS Coordinator, Randall Tobias, who coordinates not only the GHAI programs in the focus countries, but also the HIV/AIDS programs of USAID and other agencies in both focus and non-focus countries.

President Bush made AIDS a special focus of his five-day trip to Africa in July 2003. On July 10, speaking in Botswana, the President said that, "this is the deadliest enemy Africa has ever faced, and you will not face this epidemic alone." On July 8, in Senegal, the President told Africans, "we will join with you in turning the tide against AIDS in Africa." On September 22, 2003, then Secretary of State Colin Powell told a U.N. General Assembly special session on AIDS that the epidemic was "more devastating than any terrorist attack" and that the United States would "remain at the forefront" of efforts to combat the epidemic.

On February 23, 2004, the Department of State issued a report [http://www.state.gov/s/ gac/rl/or/c11652.htm] providing details on the PEPFAR initiative. At the same time, the Administration announced plans to release PEPFAR funds for treatment programs conducted by the Elizabeth Glaser Pediatric AIDS Foundation, Harvard's School of Public Health, Colombia's Mailman School of Public Health, and Catholic Relief Services.

Many AIDS activists and others have praised the President's initiatives, but critics maintain that PEPFAR in particular is getting off to a slow start and have urged increased appropriations. Some also see the program as too strongly unilateral and would like the United States to be acting in closer cooperation with other countries and donors, particularly the Global Fund to Fight AIDS, Tuberculosis, and Malaria. Some are questioning whether PEPFAR will do enough to strengthen African health care institutions and capabilities for coping with AIDS over the long term; or whether the funds will flow primarily to U.S.-based organizations.

U.N. Secretary General Kofi Annan, during an interview at the July 2004 international AIDS conference in Bangkok, urged the United States to contribute $1 billion annually to the Global Fund to Fight AIDS, Tuberculosis, and Malaria; but U.S. Global AIDS Coordinator Randall Tobias said "It's not going to happen." (For further information, see CRS Report RL31712, *The Global Fund to Fight AIDS, Tuberculosis, and Malaria: Background and Current Issues*.) Annan asked the United States to show the same leadership in the AIDS struggle that it had shown in the war on terrorism. U.S. State Department spokesman Richard Boucher rejected the implied criticism, saying that the Bush Administration had taken the AIDS crisis very seriously and that the $15 billion pledged to fight the epidemic over five years was an "enormous and significant amount." In a speech interrupted by protestors, Tobias told the conference that "At this point, perhaps the most critical mistake we can make is to allow this pandemic to divide us."

Treatment

The *Financial Times* reported in April 2004, that the United States was withholding support from a program intended to treat 140,000 AIDS patients in Kenya with antiretrovirals because the program would rely on a generic 3-drug combination (FDC) pill. Many favor approval of FDCs, including copies of drugs manufactured by different companies, on grounds that they are simpler to prescribe and need to be taken just once or twice a day. U.S. officials had expressed concerns that further study was needed to assure that their widespread or improper distribution did not contribute to the emergence of resistant HIV strains.

The issue was submitted to a panel of experts instructed to report by mid-May 2004. Several members of Congress subsequently wrote to President Bush asking that the United States join an international consensus that generics are safe and essential for the treatment of AIDS. On May 16, 2004, Health and Human Services Secretary Tommy Thompson announced that the United States Food and Drug Administration (FDA) was instituting an expedited process that could lead to the approval of the use of FDCs in programs funded by PEPFAR. Many hailed the announcement as a step forward in making cheaper and more reliable antiretroviral therapy available in Africa, but critics said it placed an unnecessary hurdle in the way of distributing such pills. They maintained that the United States should have relied on the approval process of the World Health organization, which had already cleared such pills. In January 2005, the FDA cleared the first generic FDC for use in the PEPFAR program. Manufactured by Aspen Pharmacare of South Africa, the three-drug FDC will is expected to make treatment available for $20-$30 per patient per month, compared with $55 for the three brand-name drugs. On January 28, 2005, the U.S. Government Accountability Office (GAO) issued a report (GAO-05-133) finding that the regimen of antiretroviral drugs (ARVs) offered under PEPFAR is narrower and more costly than regimens offered by other programs.

On March 23, 2005, the Department of State released *Engendering Bold Leadership: The President's Emergency Plan for AIDS Relief* (PEPFAR), the first annual report to Congress on the President's initiative. Global AIDS Coordinator Randall Tobias called PEPFAR "coordinated, accountable, and powerful," and the report stated that 152,000 patients in sub-Saharan Africa were receiving AIDS treatment as a result. According to the report, 119 million had been reached with mass media campaigns promoting abstinence and being faithful, while 71 million had been reached with messages promoting other prevention measures, including the use of condoms.

Spending

Table 2 reports available information on recent U.S. spending levels on AIDS programs in Africa. Under the FY2006 request, GHAI assistance to the 12 focus countries in sub-Saharan Africa would grow by 54% to just over $1.2 billion, or 61% or the total GHAI request. Prior to the launching of PEPFAR, USAID, and the Global AIDS Program (GAP) of the Centers for Disease Control (CDC) in the Department of Health and Human Services were the principal channels for HIV/AIDS assistance to Africa. The drop in USAID funding in Table 2 from FY2004 to FY2005 results from the shift in funds in the 12 GHAI focus countries in Africa to the Office of the Global AIDS Coordinator at the Department of State. This was done in order to simplify the budget and enhance transparency. Most USAID spending on HIV/AIDS in Africa is through the Child Survival and Health Programs Fund, but limited amounts are provided through the Economic Support Fund. Information on GAP spending in Africa for FY2004 and subsequent years is not yet available (NA) due to a change in budget structure at the Department of Health and Human Services. The Defense Department (DOD) has undertaken an HIV/AIDS education program primarily with African armed forces. As in other recent years, the Administration has not requested funding for this program in FY2006, but in FY2005 Congress continued to support it by appropriating $7.5 million. Funds from the Foreign Military Financing (FMF) program are also used to support this initiative. Meanwhile, a Department of Labor (DOL) program supports AIDS education in the workplace in four sub-Saharan countries. (For more information, see CRS Report RS21181, *HIV/AIDS International Programs: Appropriations, FY2003-FY2006*.) Additional U.S. funds reach Africa indirectly through the AIDS programs of the United Nations, the World Bank, and the Global Fund to Fight AIDS, Tuberculosis, and Malaria.

Table 2. U.S. Bilateral Spending on Fighting AIDS in Africa ($ millions)

	FY 2000	FY 2001	FY 2002	FY 2003	FY2004 Est.	FY2005 Est.	FY2006 Request
USAID	109	144	183	320	234.0	82.3	82.4
CDC (GAP)	30	77	84	107	NA	NA	NA
GHAI (State)	-	-	-	-	263.8	781.5	1,206.3
DOD	0	5	14	7	4.2	7.5	0
FMF	0	0	0	2	1.5	2.0	2.0
DOL	0	3	6	5	2.1	NA	0
Total	139	229	287	441			

The scale of the response to the pandemic in Africa by the United States and others remains a subject of intense debate. The U.N. Special Envoy for HIV/AIDS in Africa, Stephen Lewis, has been a persistent critic, telling a September 2003 conference on AIDS in Africa that he was "enraged by the behavior of the rich powers" with respect to the epidemic. The singer Bono said he had a "good old row" with President Bush in a September 16, 2003 meeting on the level of U.S. funding for fighting the international AIDS epidemic. Nonetheless, as noted above, others have argued that Africa's ability to absorb increased AIDS funding is limited and that health infrastructure will have to be expanded before new funds can be spent effectively.

Legislative Action, 2000-2004

In August 2000, the Global AIDS and Tuberculosis Relief Act of 2000 (P.L. 106-264) became law. This legislation authorized funding for fiscal years 2001 and 2002 for a comprehensive, coordinated, worldwide HIV/AIDS effort under USAID. In the 107th Congress, a number of bills were introduced with international or Africa-related HIV/AIDS related provisions. A major international AIDS authorization bill, H.R. 2069, passed both the House and Senate during the 107th Congress but did not go to conference. (For information on appropriations for HIV/AIDS programs, see CRS Report RS21114,

HIV/AIDS: Appropriations for Worldwide Programs in FY2001 and FY2002.)

In May 2003, Congress approved and President Bush signed into law H.R. 1298/ P.L. 108-25, the United States Leadership Against HIV/AIDS, Tuberculosis, and Malaria Act of 2003. This bill backs the President's Emergency Plan for AIDS Relief by authorizing $3 billion per year for FY2004 through FY2008 (a total of $15 billion) and creating the office of the Global AIDS Coordinator at the Department of State. Appropriations measures have supported a variety of programs helping Africa fight the pandemic; for further information, see CRS Report RS21181, *HIV/AIDS International Programs: Appropriations, FY2002-FY2004.*

Legislation in the 109th Congress

Bills introduced in the 109th Congress, with provisions related to the African AIDS pandemic, include the following.

- **H.R. 155 (Millender-McDonald),** Mother to Child Plus Appropriations Act for Fiscal Year 2005.
- **H.R. 164 (Millender McDonald),** International Pediatric HIV/AIDS Network Act of 2005.
- **H.R. 1409 (Lee)/S. 350 (Lugar),** Assistance for Orphans and Other Vulnerable Children in Developing Countries Act of 2005.
- **S. 850 (Frist),** Global Health Corps Act of 2005.

ENDNOTES

[1] George P. Schmid and others, "Transmission of HIV-1 Infection in Sub-Saharan Africa and Effect of Elimination of Unsafe Injections," *The Lancet*, February 7, 2004.

[2] UNAIDS, UNICEF, and U.S. Agency for International Development, *Children on the Brink*, July 2004.

[3] Maria Wawer, R. Gray, and others, "Declines in HIV Prevalence in Uganda: Not as Simple as ABC," presented at the 12th Conference on Retroviruses and Opportunistic Infections, Boston.

[4] World Health Organization, *"3 by 5" Progress Report*, December 2004. Dr. Jim Yong Kim, director of HIV/AIDS programs at the World Health Organization (WHO), said on February 22, 2005, that the campaign was struggling to attain its goal. In Africa, Botswana and Uganda would likely meet their targets, but South Africa and Nigeria were lagging behind.

[5] "Global AIDS Effort Still Short of Goal," *Boston Globe*, February 23, 2005.

[6] "Africans Outdo Americans in Following AIDS Therapy," *New York Times*, September 3, 2003.

[7] Holly Burkhalter, "Misplaced Help in the AIDS Fight," *Washington Post* op-ed, May 25, 2004.

In: Aids in Africa: A Pandemic on the Move   ISBN 1-59454-596-0
Editor: Garson J. Claton, pp. 25-42   © 2006 Nova Science Publishers, Inc.

Chapter 2

THE ECONOMIC IMPACT OF AIDS*

John Stover and Lori Bollinger
The Futures Group International *in collaboration with:*
Research Triangle Institute (RTI) and
The Centre for Development and Population Activities (CEDPA)

AIDS has the potential to create severe economic impacts in many African countries. It is different from most other diseases because it strikes people in the most productive age groups and is essentially 100 percent fatal. The effects will vary according to the severity of the AIDS epidemic and the structure of the national economies. The two major economic effects are a reduction in the labor supply and increased costs:

Labor Supply

- The loss of young adults in their most productive years will affect overall economic output
- If AIDS is more prevalent among the economic elite, then the impact may be much larger than the absolute number of AIDS deaths indicates

* POLICY is a five-year project funded by the U.S. Agency for International Development under Contract No. CCP-C-00-95-00023-04, beginning September 1, 1995. The project is implemented by The Futures Group International in collaboration with Research Triangle Institute (RTI) and The Centre for Development and Population Activities (CEDPA).

Costs

- The direct costs of AIDS include expenditures for medical care, drugs, and funeral expenses
- Indirect costs include lost time due to illness, recruitment and training costs to replace workers, and care of orphans
- If costs are financed out of savings, then the reduction in investment could lead to a significant reduction in economic growth

A World Bank study of the economic impacts of AIDS in Africa concluded that the macroeconomic impacts of AIDS could be significant.[1] Yet there is still time to mitigate the economic impact of AIDS; over half of Africa's population live in countries where the epidemic is "concentrated," that is, where HIV infection is concentrated in groups with risky behavior and is not yet widespread in the general population.[2]

The economic effects of AIDS will be felt first by individuals and their families, then ripple outwards to firms and businesses and the macroeconomy. This paper will consider each of these levels in turn and provide examples from various African countries to illustrate these impacts.

ECONOMIC IMPACT OF AIDS ON HOUSEHOLDS

The household impacts begin as soon as a member of the household starts to suffer from HIV-related illnesses:

- Loss of income of the patient (who is frequently the main breadwinner)
- Household expenditures for medical expenses may increase substantially
- Other members of the household, usually daughters and wives, may miss school or work less in order to care for the sick person

---

[1] Over, M. 1992. The Macroeconomic Impact of AIDS in Sub-Saharan Africa. AFTPN Technical Working Paper 3. World Bank, Africa Technical Department, Population, Health, and Nutrition Division, Washington, DC.

[2] Ainsworth, M and M Over. 1998. AIDS and Development: The Role of Government. AIDS; 12(5): 12-13. IAS Newsletter No. 9.

- Death results in: a permanent loss of income, from less labor on the farm or from lower remittances; funeral and mourning costs; and the removal of children from school in order to save on educational expenses and increase household labor, resulting in a severe loss of future earning potential.

Funeral and Health Care Expenditures
Increase When an Adult in the Household Dies

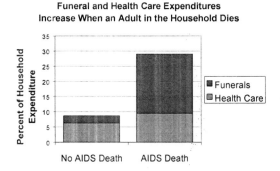

Studies in Tanzania, Cote d'Ivoire, Uganda, and Ethiopia have documented the tremendous burden of loss of income, large health care expenditures, and consumption of savings to pay for funeral and mourning costs:

- In **Tanzania**, a study of adult mortality found that 8 percent of total household expenditure went to medical care and funerals in households that had an adult death in the preceding 12 months. In households with no adult death the figure was only 0.8 percent. In addition to increased expenditures, many households experienced a reduction in remittances if the adult member worked outside the home. In partial compensation for these financial setbacks, many households were forced to remove children from school in order to reduce education-related expenditures and have the children help with household chores.[3]
- In **Cote d'Ivoire**, households with an HIV/AIDS patient spent twice as much on medical expenses as other households. Furthermore, 80 percent of the expenditures went to the AIDS patient, rather than to other household members who are ill. When

---

[3] Mead Over, Martha Ainsworth, et al. 1996. Coping with AIDS: The Economic Impact of Adult Mortality from AIDS and Other Causes on Households in Kagera, Tanzania.

the person with AIDS died or moved away, average consumption fell by as much as 44 percent during the following year.[4]

- In **Uganda**, the economic impact of HIV-related deaths was stronger than other types of death, as households lost much of their savings in order to pay health care and funeral expenditures. Asset ownership declined when the death of an HIV+ member occured, but remained stable when the death was of an HIV- member.[5]
- In **Ethiopia**, a study of 25 AIDS-afflicted rural families found that the average cost of treatment, funeral and mourning expenses amounted to several times the average household income.[6]

ECONOMIC IMPACT OF AIDS ON AGRICULTURE

Agriculture is the largest sector in most African economies accounting for a large portion of production and a majority of employment. Studies done in Tanzania and other countries have shown that AIDS will have adverse effects on agriculture, including loss of labor supply and remittance income. The loss of a few workers at the crucial periods of planting and harvesting can significantly reduce the size of the harvest. In countries where food security has been a continuous issue because of drought, any declines in household production can have serious consequences. Additionally, a loss of agricultural labor is likely to cause farmers to switch to less-labor-intensive crops. In many cases this may mean switching from export crops to food crops.[7] Thus, AIDS could affect the production of cash crops as well as food crops.

---

[4] Bechu, N. 1998. The impact of AIDS on the economy of families in Cote d'Ivoire: Changes in consumption among AIDS-affected households. In M Ainsworth, L Fransen, and M Over, eds., Confronting AIDS: Evidence from the developing world: Selected background papers for the World Bank Policy Research Report. European Commission: United Kingdom; and AIDS Analysis Africa; 8(1): 2-3

[5] Menon, R, MJ Wawer, JK Konde-Lule, NK Sewankambo, and C Li. 1998. The economic impact of adult mortality on households in Rakai district, Uganda. In M Ainsworth, L Fransen, and M Over, eds., Confronting AIDS: Evidence from the developing world: Selected background papers for the World Bank Policy Research Report. European Commission: United Kingdom

[6] Demeke, M. 1993. The Potential Impact of HIV/AIDS on the Rural Sector of Ethiopia. Unpublished manuscript, January 1993.

[7] Ilinigumugabo, A. 1996. The economic consequences of AIDS in Africa. African Journal of Fertility, Sexuality and Reproductive Health; 1(2):153-61.

Reduction in Marketed Output Due to AIDS Deaths in Zimbabwe

Crops	Reduction in Marketed Output
Maize	61%
Cotton	47%
Vegetables	49%
Groundnuts	37%
Cattle Owned	29%

- A study done by the **Zimbabwe** Farmers Union (ZFU) showed that the death of a breadwinner due to AIDS will cut the marketed output of maize in small scale farming and communal areas by 61 percent. Similar results were obtained for other crops (see table at right). The fall in marketed output results from losses of labor and remittances and the need to spend scarce resources on medical expenses.[8]

- In **Ethiopia**, the male head of the household is responsible for special tasks, such as oxen cultivation, harvesting, threshing and farm management. One study found that the effect of an AIDS death varied by region: it would have the most severe effect on harvesting teff in Nazareth, on digging holes for transplanting enset plants in Atat, on ploughing millet fields in Baherdar, and on picking coffee in Yirgalem. Women are generally responsible for other tasks: leveling, weeding, harvesting minor crops, transporting produce, and household duties. The death of the wife to AIDS can make it difficult for other household members to carry out these tasks, in addition to caring for children. The death of a family member because of AIDS also leads to a reduction in savings and investment. The stock of food grain can be depleted to provide food for mourners and the other expenses were met most often by selling livestock. Such loss of productive assets only makes it harder to survive in the future.[9]

- In Kagabiro village, **Tanzania**, when a household contained an AIDS patient, the household labor supply was severely affected: on average, 29% of household labor was spent on AIDS-related

---

[8] Kwaramba, P (1997) "The Socio-Economic Impact of HIV/AIDS on Communal Agricultural Systems in Zimbabwe," Zimbabwe Farmers Union, Friedrich Ebert Stiftung Economic Advisory Project, Working Paper 19, Harare, Zimbabwe.

matters, including care of the patient and funeral duties. If two people were devoted to nursing duties, as occurred in 66% of the cases, the total labor loss was 43%, on average.[10]

- In **Malawi**, 10% of GDP comes from estate agriculture. A recent study evaluated the costs of HIV/AIDS on a tea estate there (see table at right). The study found that the costs are determined by the levels of both employee benefits and of skilled labor necessary for production. It predicted that, in the longer term, the negative impact on the supply of skilled labor will be the strongest effect of HIV/AIDS.[11] It will become increasingly difficult to recruit skilled people, even at the national level.

- Data collected in **Uganda** indicate that agricultural tasks were frequently disrupted when women needed to care for household members ill with AIDS-related conditions.[12]

Cost of HIV/AIDS on a Tea Estate in Malawi

Description	Total Cost (£)	Related to HIV (%)	Cost of HIV (£)
Provision of medical services	22,275	25	5,569
Funeral costs	928	75	696
Death in service benefits	4,691	100	4,691
Absence	14,875	25	3,719
Total	42,769		14,675

[9] Demeke, M. 1993. The Potential Impact of HIV/AIDS on the Rural Sector of Ethiopia. Unpublished manuscript, January 1993.

[10] Tibaijuka, AK. 1997. AIDS and Economic Welfare in Peasant Agriculture: Case Studies from Kagabiro Village, Kagera Region, Tanzania. World Development; 25(6):963-975.

[11] Jones, C. 1997. What HIV cost a tea estate in Malawi. AIDS Analysis Africa; 7(3): 5-7.

[12] Taylor, L, J Seeley, E Kajura. 1996. Informal care for illness in rural southwest Uganda: the central role that women play. Health Transition Review; 6(1):49-56.

ECONOMIC IMPACT OF AIDS ON FIRMS

AIDS may have a significant impact on some firms. AIDS-related illnesses and deaths to employees affect a firm by both increasing expenditures and reducing revenues. Expenditures are increased for health care costs, burial fees and training and recruitment of replacement employees. Revenues may be decreased because of absenteeism due to illness or attendance at funerals and time spent on training. Labor turnover can lead to a less experienced labor force that is less productive.

Factors Leading to Increased Expenditure	Factors Leading to Decreased Revenue
Health care costs	Absenteeism due to illness
Burial fees	Time off to attend funerals
Training and recruitment	Time spent on training
	Labor turnover

Distribution of Increased Labour Costs Due to HIV/AIDS in in Selected Firms in Kenya and Botswana

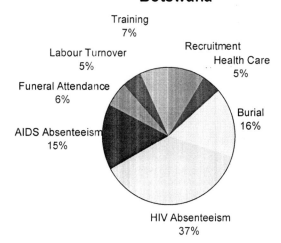

Training
7%

Labour Turnover
5%

Funeral Attendance
6%

AIDS Absenteeism
15%

Recruitment
Health Care
5%

Burial
16%

HIV Absenteeism
37%

The actual distribution of these costs has been calculated as part of various USAID-funded AIDSCAP studies of the private sector impact of AIDS:

- One study examining several firms in **Botswana** and **Kenya** showed that the most significant factors in increased labor costs were absenteeism due to HIV or AIDS and increased burial costs as shown in the figure to the right.[13]

- Another study in **Zimbabwe** found that the major expense was health care costs. The transport company in this study has a large staff of 11,500 workers. Since the company offers significant health benefits to its employees, the cost of AIDS is even higher than for other companies that do not provide such benefits. The study estimated that there are currently more than 3,400 workers who are infected with HIV and 64 who died from AIDS in 1996. The total costs of AIDS to the company in 1996 were estimated at Z$39 million, equal to about 20 percent of the company's profits. More than half of this amount resulted from increased health care costs. By 2005 the cost of AIDS to the company could reach Z$108 million. There may be indirect costs as well. The report speculates that HIV/AIDS will worsen employee morale and create greater labor-management tensions and cause a labor shortage among skilled positions.[14]

Various studies have also examined the total annual cost of AIDS to different companies, as well as the annual cost of AIDS per employee.[15] These studies found that the annual cost of AIDS per employee varied from US$17 to US$300, as shown in the following table:

---

[13] Roberts, Matthew and Bill Rau, African Workplace Profiles: Private Sector AIDS Policy, AIDSCAP, Arlington, VA, USA.

[14] Roberts, Matthew and Bill Rau, African Workplace Profiles: Private Sector AIDS Policy, AIDSCAP, Arlington, VA, USA

[15] Roberts, Matthew and Bill Rau, African Workplace Profiles: Private Sector AIDS Policy, AIDSCAP, Arlington, VA, USA.; Aventin, L and P Huard. 1997. HIV/AIDS and manufacturing in Abidjan. *AIDS Analysis Africa*, Vol 7(3): June 1997.; Ainsworth, Martha, "The Impact of HIV/AIDS on African Development", presented at the African Development Bank HIV/AIDS and Development in Africa Symposium, May 11, 1993.

Company Name	Total Annual Cost of AIDS	Annual Cost of AIDS per Employee
Botswana Diamond Valuing	US$ 125,941	US$ 237
Botswana Meat Commission	US$ 370,200	US$ 268
Cote d'Ivoire food processing firm	US$ 33,207	US$ 120
Cote d'Ivoire textile firm	US$ 32,667	US$ 29
Cote d'Ivoire packaging firm	US$ 10,398	US$ 125
Kenyan automobile firm	US$ 21,312	US$ 17
Kenyan transport firm	US$ 61,132	US$ 28
Muhoroni Sugar, Kenya	US$ 58,303	US$ 49
Kenyan lumber firm	US$ 40,630	US$ 25
Uganda Railway Corporation	US$ 77,000	US$ 300

Increased labor costs can reduce the profits necessary for expansion. This impact on profits can be considerable:

- The Indeni Petroleum Refinery in **Zambia** spent US$26,400 on AIDS-related costs in 1994, more than its declared profits of US$25,514 in that year.[16]
- A study in **South Africa** examined the expected impact of AIDS on employee benefits, and thus on corporate profits. It found that at current levels of benefits per employee, the total costs of benefits would rise from 7 percent of salaries in 1995 to 19 percent by 2005. Since these additional costs will have to be paid at the same time that productivity is declining, due to AIDS, the net impact on profits could be significant.[17]

Finally, other costs associated with AIDS that firms face include:

- The **Uganda** Railway Corporation has been hard hit by AIDS among it employees, experiencing a labor turnover rate of 15 percent per year in recent years.[18]
- Medical aid companies in **Zimbabwe** have estimated that meeting all the claims of just one percent of HIV-infected members could

[16] Southern African Economist, 1997. "AIDS toll on regional economies," April 15-May 15, 1997.

[17] Southern African Economist, 1997. "AIDS toll on regional economies," April 15-May 15, 1997.

[18] Ainsworth, Martha, "The Impact of HIV/AIDS on African Development", presented at the African Development Bank HIV/AIDS and Development in Africa Symposium, May 11, 1993.

result in a 31 percent increase in insurance rates. Most of this increase would have to be paid by employers.[19]

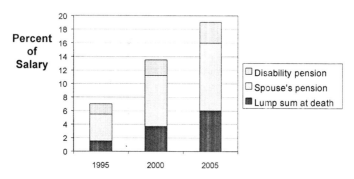

Illustrative Impact of AIDS on Employee Benefits in South Africa

For some smaller firms the loss of one or more key employees could be catastrophic, leading to the collapse of the firm. In others, the impact may be small. Firms in some key sectors, such as transportation and mining, are likely to suffer larger impacts than firms in other sectors. In poorly managed situations the HIV-related costs to companies can be high. However, with proactive management these costs can be mitigated through effective prevention and management strategies.

IMPACTS ON OTHER ECONOMIC SECTORS

AIDS will also have significant effects in other key sectors. Among them are health, transport, mining, education and water.

- **Health.** AIDS will affect the health sector for two reasons: (1) it will increase the number of people seeking services and (2) health care for AIDS patients is more expensive than for most other conditions. The number of AIDS patients seeking care is already overwhelming health care systems. In many hospitals in Africa, half of hospital beds are now occupied by AIDS patients. AIDS is also an expensive disease. The graph shows projected expenditure on

---

[19] Southern African Economist, 1997. "AIDS toll on regional economies," April 15-May 15, 1997.

AIDS as a percentage of public health spending for three African countries.[20] On average, treating an AIDS patient for one year is about as expensive as educating ten primary school students for one year. Governments will face trade-offs along at least three dimensions: treating AIDS versus preventing HIV infection; treating AIDS versus treating other illnesses; and spending for health versus spending for other objectives. Maintaining a healthy population is an important goal in its own right and is crucial to the development of a productive workforce essential for economic development.

Potential AIDS Treatment Costs as a Perent of the Ministry of Health Budget

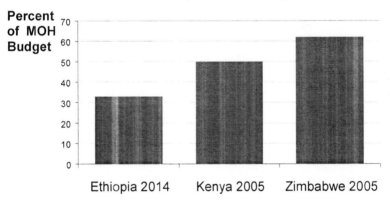

- **Transport.** The transport sector is especially vulnerable to AIDS and important to AIDS prevention. Building and maintaining transport infrastructure often involves sending teams of men away from their families for extended periods of time, increasing the likelihood of multiple sexual partners. The people who operate transport services (truck drivers, train crews, sailors) spend many days and nights away from their families. A survey of bus and truck drivers in Cameroon found that they spent an average of 14 days away from home on each trip and that 68 percent had sex during the

[20] Ministry of Health, 1998. *AIDS in Ethiopia, Second Edition*, Addis Ababa: Epidemiology and AIDS Department, 1998.; NASCOP, 1998. *AIDS in Kenya, Fourth Edition*. Nairobi: National AIDS and STDs Control Programme, 1998.; Ministry of Health and Child Welfare, 1998. *HIV/AIDS in Zimbabwe*. Harare: National AIDS Coordination Programme, 1998.

most recent trip and 25 percent had sex every night they were away.[21] Most transport managers are highly trained professionals who are hard to replace if they die. Governments face the dilemma of improving transport as an essential element of national development while protecting the health of the workers and their families.

- **Mining.** The mining sector is a key source of foreign exchange for many countries. Most mining is conducted at sites far from population centers forcing workers to live apart from their families for extended periods of time. They often resort to commercial sex. Many become infected with HIV and spread that infection to their spouses and communities when they return home. Highly trained mining engineers can be very difficult to replace. As a result, a severe AIDS epidemic can seriously threaten mine production.

- **Education.** AIDS affects the education sector in at least three ways: the supply of experienced teachers will be reduced by AIDS-related illness and death; children may be kept out of school if they are needed at home to care for sick family members or to work in the fields; and children may drop out of school if their families can not afford school fees due to reduced household income as a result of an AIDS death. Another problem is that teenage children are especially susceptible to HIV infection. Therefore, the education system also faces a special challenge to educate students about AIDS and equip them to protect themselves.

- **Water.** Developing water resources in arid areas and controlling excess water during rainy periods requires highly skilled water engineers and constant maintenance of wells, dams, embankments, etc. The loss of even a small number of highly trained engineers can place entire water systems and significant investment at risk. These engineers may be especially susceptible to HIV because of the need to spend many nights away from their families.

MACROECONOMIC IMPACT OF AIDS

The macroeconomic impact of AIDS is difficult to assess. Most studies have found that estimates of the macroeconomic impacts are sensitive to assumptions about how AIDS affects savings and investment rates and

---

[21] *AIDS Analysis Africa*, Vol. 4 (5), September/October 1994.

whether AIDS affects the best-educated employees more than others. Few studies have been able to incorporate the impacts at the household and firm level in macroeconomic projections. Some studies have found that the impacts may be small, especially if there is a plentiful supply of excess labor and worker benefits are small. Other studies have found significant macroeconomic impacts. Studies in Tanzania, Cameroon, Zambia, Swaziland, Kenya and other sub-Saharan African countries have found that the rate of economic growth could be reduced by as much as 25 percent over a 20-year period.

There are several mechanisms by which AIDS affects macroeconomic performance.

- AIDS deaths lead directly to a reduction in the number of workers available. These deaths occur to workers in their most productive years. As younger, less experienced workers replace these experienced workers, worker productivity is reduced. The graph to the right illustrates the magnitude of the problem in five African countries.[22] It shows the increase in mortality among men of working age from the late 1980s to the mid-1990s. Most, if not all, of this increase is due to AIDS.

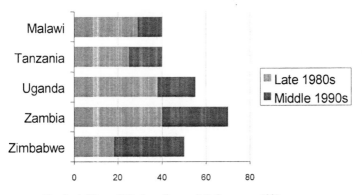

Increase in Mortality Among Men 15-60

Probability of Dying from All Causes (%)

---

[22] UNAIDS, 1998. *Report on the global HIV/AIDS epidemic, June 1998*. Geneva: UNAIDS, WHO,. 1998.

- A shortage of workers leads to higher wages, which leads to higher domestic production costs. Higher production costs lead to a loss of international competitiveness which can cause foreign exchange shortages.
- Lower government revenues and reduced private savings (because of greater health care expenditures and a loss of worker income) can cause a significant drop in savings and capital accumulation. This leads to slower employment creation in the formal sector, which is particularly capital intensive.
- Reduced worker productivity and investment leads to fewer jobs in the formal sector. As a result some workers will be pushed from high paying jobs in the formal sector to lower paying jobs in the informal sector.
- The overall impact of AIDS on the macro-economy is small at first but increases significantly over time.

Several studies have found that these effects could be large in some African countries.

- A World Bank study examined the macroeconomic impact of AIDS in 30 sub-Saharan African countries.[23] This study concluded that the net effect is likely to be a reduction of the annual growth rate of GDP of 0.8 to 1.4 percentage points per year and a 0.3 percentage point reduction in the annual growth rate of GDP per capita.
- A simulation model of the economy of **Cameroon** concluded that the annual growth rate of GDP could have been reduced by as much as 2 percentage points during the 1987-1991 period because of AIDS.[24]
- A study of the macroeconomic impacts of AIDS in **Zambia** found that by 2000 the GDP would be 5 to 10 percent lower because of AIDS than it would be if there were no AIDS affecting the population. The authors concluded, *"...without unprecedented*

---

[23] Over, Mead, 1992. "The Macroeconomic impact of AIDS in Sub-Saharan Africa," The World Bank, Technical Working Paper No. 3., 1992.

[24] Kambou, Gerard, Shantayanan Deverajan and Mead Over. 1992. "The Economic Impact of AIDS in an African Country: Simulations with a Computable General Equilibrium Model of Cameroon", *Journal of African Economies*, Volume 1, Number 1.

infusions of free foreign aid to mitigate the effects of AIDS, the economy of Zambia will suffer considerable damage. "[25]

Percent Reduction in Future GDP due to AIDS

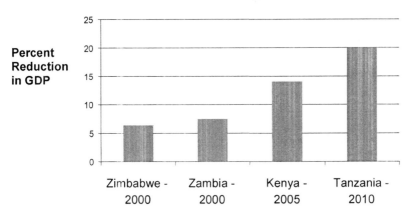

- An assessment of the macroeconomic impacts of AIDS in **Tanzania** by the Government of Tanzania, the World Bank and the World Health Organization in 1991 found that total GDP will be 15 to 25 percent smaller in 2010 because of the impact of AIDS.[26]
- A study of the impact of AIDS on the economy of **Kenya** projected that GDP will be 14 percent lower in 2005 than it would have been without AIDS. GDP per capita will be 10 percent less in 2005.[27]

WHAT CAN BE DONE?

AIDS has the potential to cause severe deterioration in the economic conditions of many countries. However, this is not inevitable. There is much that can be done now to keep the epidemic from getting worse and to mitigate the negative effects. Among the responses that are necessary are:

[25] Forgy, Larry. 1993. "Mitigating AIDS: The Economic Impacts of AIDS inZambia and Measures to Counter Them," REDSO/ESA, February 1993.
[26] Cuddington, JT, 1992. Modelling the Macroeconomic Effects of AIDS, with an Application to Tanzania, *World Bank Economic Review*, 7(2):172-189.
[27] Hancock, John; David Nalo; Monica Aoko; Roselyn Mutemi; Steven Forsythe, 1996. "The Macroeconomic Impacts of AIDS," *AIDS in Kenya*, FHI: Washington, DC, 1996.

- **Prevent new infections.** The most effective response will be to support programs to reduce the number of new infections in the future. After more than a decade of research and pilot programs, we now know how to prevent most new infections. An effective national response should include information, education and communications; voluntary counseling and testing; condom promotion and availability; expanded and improved services to prevent and treat sexually transmitted diseases; and efforts to protect human rights and reduce stigma and discrimination. Governments, NGOs and the commercial sector, working together in a multi-sectoral effort can make a difference. Workplace-based programs can prevent new infections among experienced workers.
- **Design major development projects appropriately.** Some major development activities may inadvertently facilitate the spread of HIV. Major construction projects often require large numbers of male workers to live apart from their families for extended periods of time, leading to increased opportunities for commercial sex. A World Bank-funded pipeline construction project in Cameroon was redesigned to avoid this problem by creating special villages where workers could live with their families. Special prevention programs can be put in place from the very beginning in projects such as mines or new ports where commercial sex might be expected to flourish.
- **Programs to address specific problems.** Special programs can mitigate the impact of AIDS by addressing some of the most severe problems. Reduced school fees can help children from poor families and AIDS orphans stay in school longer and avoid deterioration in the education level of the workforce. Tax benefits or other incentives for training can encourage firms to maintain worker productivity in spite of the loss of experienced workers.
- **Mitigate the effects of AIDS on poverty.** The impacts of AIDS on households can be reduced to some extent by publicly funded programs to address the most severe problems. Such programs have included home care for people with HIV/AIDS, support for the basic needs of the households coping with AIDS, foster care for AIDS orphans, food programs for children and support for educational expenses. Such programs can help families and particularly children survive some of the consequences of an adult AIDS death that occur when families are poor or become poor as a

result of the costs of AIDS. The costs of these programs can vary widely.[28]

Annual Costs of Programmes to Mitigate the Household Impacts of AIDS, Kagera, Tanzania, 1992

Type of Programme	Annual Cost (US$)
Home care for people with AIDS	$227 per patient
Orphanage care	$1,063 per child
Foster care	$185 per child
Feeding post	$69 per child
Basic needs support	$47 per household
Educational support	$13 per child

A strong political commitment to the fight against AIDS is crucial. Countries that have shown the most success, such as Uganda, Thailand and Senegal, all have strong support from the top political leaders. This support is critical for several reasons. First, it sets the stage for an open approach to AIDS that helps to reduce the stigma and discrimination that often hamper prevention efforts. Second, it facilitates a multi-sectoral approach by making it clear that the fight against AIDS is a national priority. Third, it signals to individuals and community organizations involved in the AIDS programs that their efforts are appreciated and valued. Finally, it ensures that the program will receive an appropriate share of national and international donor resources to fund important programs.

Perhaps the most important role for the government in the fight against AIDS is to ensure an open and supportive environment for effective programs. Governments need to make AIDS a national priority, not a problem to be avoided. By stimulating and supporting a broad multi-sectoral approach that includes all segments of society, governments can create the conditions in which prevention, care and mitigation programs can succeed and protect the country's future development prospects.

---

[28] World Bank, 1997. *Confronting AIDS: Public Priorities in a Global Epidemic.* New York: Oxford University Press.

In: Aids in Africa: A Pandemic on the Move   ISBN 1-59454-596-0
Editor: Garson J. Claton, pp. 43-69   © 2006 Nova Science Publishers, Inc.

Chapter 3

BIBLIOGRAPHY–BOOKS

Achineku, I. The AIDS crisis in Africa: our Christian responsibiblity / I. Achineku & Map International. Published/Created: Potchefstroom: Institute for Reformational Studies , 1999 . Description: 44 p. ISBN: 1868223507. Series: Studiestuk; 380. LC Classification: African Section Pamphlet Coll

Africa today. (Agricultural Aids Foundation). Current Frequency: Unknown. Notes: Holdings in 3x5 file.

AIDS & society. Published/Created: Hanover, NH: African-Caribbean Institute, c1989-1995. Related Authors: African-Caribbean Institute (Hanover, N.H.) International Development Research Centre (Canada) United States. Bureau of the Census. Description: 6

v.; 28 cm. Vol. 1, no. 1 (Oct. 1989)-v. 6, no. 4 (July/Aug. 1995). Current Frequency: Quarterly Absrb'd in part by: AIDS analysis Asia (DLC)sn 95050345 (OCoLC)33860934 AIDS analysis Africa (London, England) (DLC)sn 96039030 (OCoLC)27021673 ISSN: 1055-0380. Notes: Title from caption. Issues for <Apr./May 1991- include inserts from the International Development Research Centre of Canada and the U.S. Bureau of the Census. SERBIB/SERLOC merged record. Subjects: AIDS (Disease)--Social aspects--Periodicals. AIDS (Disease)--Government policy--Periodicals. Acquired Immunodeficiency Syndrome--epidemiology periodicals. Acquired Immunodeficiency Syndrome--prevention & control periodicals. HIV Infections--

epidemiology--periodicals. HIV Infections--prevention & control--periodicals. LC Classification: RA644.A25 A287. Dewey Class No.: 362.1/9697/92 2 20

AIDS analysis Africa. Edition Information: Southern Africa ed. Published/Created: Rivonia, South Africa: Aids Policy Research Group and Pro Bono Medica Medica Publishers Ltd, [1990-. Related Authors: Aids Policy Research Group (South Africa). Description: v.; 29 cm. Vol. 1, no. 1 (June/July 1990)-. Current Frequency: Bimonthly ISSN: 1016-4731. Notes: Title from caption. SERBIB/SERLOC merged record. Subjects: AIDS (Disease)--Africa, Southern--Periodicals. LC Classification: RA644.A25 A3322. Dewey Class No.: 362.1/969792/0096805 20

AIDS and associated cancers in Africa: 2nd international symposium, Naples, October 7-9, 1987 / editors, G. Giraldo ... [et al.]. Published/Created: Basel; New York: Karger, c1988. Related Authors: Giraldo, G. (Gaetano) World Health Organization. International Symposium on AIDS and Associated Cancers in Africa (2nd: 1987: Naples,

Italy). Description: x, 346 p.: ill.; 25 cm. ISBN: 3805547013 Notes: Based on the Second International Symposium on AIDS and Associated Cancers in Africa. Symposium sponsored by the World Health Organization and others. Includes bibliographies and index. Subjects: AIDS (Disease)--Africa--Epidemiology--Congresses. HIV (Viruses)--Africa--Congresses. Kaposi's sarcoma--Africa--Congresses. Acquired Immunodeficiency Syndrome--occurrence--Africa congresses. Opportunistic Infections--occurrence--Africa--Congresses. Sarcoma, Kaposi's--occurrence--Africa--congresses. LC Classification: RA644.A25 A34 1988 Dewey Class No.: 614.5/993 19

AIDS and development in Africa: a social science perspective / Kempe Ronald Hope, editor. Published/Created: New York: Haworth Press, c1999. Related Authors: Hope, Kempe R. Description: xvi, 224 p.; 23 cm. ISBN: 0789006383 (alk. paper) Notes: Includes bibliographical references and index. Subjects: AIDS (Disease)--Social aspects--Africa, Sub-Saharan. HIV infections--Social aspects--Africa, Sub-Saharan. Series: Haworth psychosocial issues of

HIV/AIDS LC Classification: RA644.A25 A3435 1999 Dewey Class No.: 362.1/969792/00967 21

AIDS and the demography of Africa / Department for Economic and Social Information and Policy Analysis. Published/Created: New York: United Nations, 1994. Related Authors: United Nations. Dept. for Economic and Social Information and Policy Analysis. Description: x, 72 p.: ill.; 28 cm. ISBN: 9211512689 Notes: "United Nations publication. Sales No. E.94.XIII.11"--t.p. verso. Includes bibliographical references (p. 69-72). Subjects: AIDS (Disease)--Africa, Sub-Saharan. LC Classification: RA644.A25 A3529 1994 Dewey Class No.: 614.5/993 20 Govt. Doc. No.: ST/ESA/Ser.A/137

AIDS in Africa / Albert E. Gunn ... [et al.]. Published/Created: Washington, D.C. (2300 N. St., N.W., Washington 20037): Foundation for Africa's Future, [1988] Related Authors: Gunn, Albert E. Foundation for Africa's Future (Alexandria, Va.). Description: 49, [10] leaves; 28 cm. Notes: "February 1988." Bibliography: leaves [3]-[10] (2nd group) Subjects: AIDS (Disease)--

Africa. LC Classification: RA644.A25 A3634 1988 Dewey Class No.: 614.5/993 20

AIDS in Africa: a manual for physicians / Peter Piot ... [et al.]. Published/Created: Geneva: World Health Organization, 1992. Related Authors: Piot, Peter, 1949- World Health Organization. Description: viii, 125 p.: ill. (some col.); 24 cm. ISBN: 924154435X Notes: Includes bibliographical references. Subjects: AIDS (Disease)--Africa. HIV Infections--diagnosis. HIV Infections--epidemiology--Africa. HIV Infections--therapy. LC Classification: RC607.A26 A34739 1992 Dewey Class No.: 616.97/92/0096 20

AIDS in Africa and the Caribbean, / edited by George C. Bond ... [et al.]. Published/Created: Boulder, Colo.: Westview Press, 1997. Related Authors: Bond, George C. Description: xv, 234 p.; 24 cm. ISBN: 0813328780 (HC) 0813328799 (PB) Notes: Based on a conference held in New York in November 1991. Includes bibliographical references (p. 195-217) and index. Subjects: AIDS (Disease)--Caribbean Area. AIDS (Disease)--Africa. Medical anthropology--Caribbean Area. Medical

anthropology--Africa. LC
Classification: RA644.A25
A36346 1997 Dewey Class
No.: 614.5/99392/096 21

AIDS in Africa: the social and
policy impact / Norman Miller
and Richard Rockwell, editors.
Published/Created: Lewiston:
Edwin Mellen Press, c1988.
Related Authors: Miller,
Norman N., 1933- Rockwell,
Richard C. Description: xxxi,
336 p.: ill.; 24 cm. ISBN:
0889461872 Notes: "Published
in association with the National
Council for International Health
... [and] the African-Caribbean
Institute"--Verso t.p. Includes
bibliographies. Subjects: AIDS
(Disease)--Africa. AIDS
(Disease)--Social aspects--
Africa. AIDS (Disease)--Africa-
-Epidemiology. Series: Studies
in African health and medicine;
v. 1. Variant Series: Studies in
African health and medicine; v.
10 [i.e. 1] LC Classification:
RA644.A25 A3635 1988
Dewey Class No.:
362.1/9697/920096 19

Aids in South Africa: the
demographic and economic
implications / The Centre for
Health Policy, Department of
Community Health, Medical
School, University of the
Witwatersrand, Johannesburg.
Published/Created:

Johannesburg: The Centre:
Thorold's Africana Books
[distributor], 1991. Related
Authors: Doyle, Peter R.
University of Witwatersrand.
Centre for Health Policy.
Description: 74 p.: ill.; 30 cm.
ISBN: 1874856397 Notes: part
I. The Impact of aids on the
South African population / Peter
R. Doyle -- part II. The
Economic impact of aids in
South Africa / Jonathan
Broomberg ... [et al.]. Includes
bibliographical references.
Subjects: AIDS (Disease)--
South Africa--Epidemiology.
AIDS (Disease)--South Africa--
Statistics. AIDS (Disease)--
Economic aspects--South
Africa. Series: Paper
(University of Witwatersrand.
Centre for Health Policy); no.
23. Variant Series: Paper; no.
23 LC Classification:
RA644.A25 A363543 1991
Dewey Class No.:
362.1/969792/00968 20

AIDS NGOs Network in East
Africa. Annual report / AIDS
NGOs Network in East Africa
(ANNEA). Published/Created:
Arusha [Tanzania]: ANNEA.
Description: v.; 30 cm. Current
Frequency: Annual Notes:
Description based on: 1996.
Subjects: AIDS NGOs Network
in East Africa--Periodicals.
Non-governmental

organizations--Africa, Eastern Periodicals. AIDS (Disease)--Africa, East--Periodicals. LC Classification: RA644.A25 A3647635a

Aids, sexuality and gender in Africa: collective strategies and struggles in Tanzania and Zambia / Carolyn Baylies and Janet Bujra [editors]; with the Gender and AIDS Group. Published/Created: New York: Routledge, 2000. Projected Pub. Date: 0012 Related Authors: Baylies, Carolyn L. (Carolyn Louise), 1947- Bujra, Janet M. Description: p. cm. ISBN: 1841420247 (hc) 1841420271 (pbk.) Notes: Includes bibliographical references and index. Subjects: AIDS (Disease)--Tanzania. AIDS (Disease)--Zambia. Series: Social aspects of AIDS LC Classification: RA644.A25 A37636 2000 Dewey Class No.: 362.1/969792/009678 21

AIDS link: AIDS health promotion in eastern, central, and southern Africa. Published/Created: Arusha, Tanzania: AIDS Regional Health Promotion Resource Centre for Eastern, Central, and Southern Africa at CEDHA, Related Authors: AIDS Regional Health Promotion Resource Centre for Eastern, Central, and Southern

Africa. Description: v.: ill.; 28 cm. Current Frequency: Quarterly Notes: Description based on: No. 2 (Mar. 1991); title from caption. SERBIB/SERLOC merged record Subjects: AIDS (Disease)--Africa, Eastern--Periodicals. AIDS (Disease)--Africa, Southern--Periodicals. AIDS (Disease)--Africa, Central--Periodicals. LC Classification: RA644.A25 A396 Dewey Class No.: 362.1/969792/009605 20

Akeroyd, Anne V. Some gendered and occupational aspects of HIV and Aids in eastern and southern Africa: changes, continuities and issues for further consideration at the end of the first decade / Anne V. Akeroyd. Published/Created: [Edinburgh]: Centre of African Studies, Edinburgh University, 1996. Description: 90 p.; 21 cm. Series: Occasional papers (University of Edinburgh, Centre of African Studies); no 60. Variant Series: Occasional papers / Centre of African Studies, Edinburgh University; no. 60 LC Classification: MLCS 99/3833 (R)

Anarfi, John Kwasi. HIV/AIDS in sub-Saharan Africa: demographic and socio-economic implications / by John

Kwasi Anarfi. Published/Created: Nairobi, Kenya: African Population and Environment Institute with assistance from Japan International Cooperation Agency, Population Education Promotion Project, [1994]. Description: 38, [1] p.: ill., map; 21 cm. Cancelled ISBN: 99669920: Notes: "November 1994." Includes bibliographical references (p. 32-[39]). Subjects: AIDS (Disease)--Africa, Sub-Saharan. Series: African population paper series; no. 3 LC Classification: RA644.A25 A49 1994 Dewey Class No.: 362.1/969792/00967 20

Baitu Rwelamira, Juvenalis. AIDS pandemic in East Africa: a moral response / Juvenalis Baitu Rwelamira. Edition Information: Rev. ed. Published/Created: [Nairobi: s.n.], 1999 (Nairobi, Kenya: CUEA Publications). Description: 43 p.; 21 cm. Cancelled ISBN: 9966902214 Notes: Includes bibliographical references. Subjects: AIDS (Disease)--Africa, East--Prevention. AIDS (Disease)--Moral and ethical aspects. Safe sex in AIDS prevention--Moral and ethical aspects. LC Classification: RA643.86.A353 B35 1999 Dewey Class No.:

362.1/969792/009676 21

Barnett, Tony. AIDS in Africa: its present and future impact / Tony Barnett and Piers Blaikie. Published/Created: New York: Guilford Press, c1992. Related Authors: Blaikie, Piers M. Description: ix, 193 p.: ill., maps; 23 cm. ISBN: 0898628806 (acid-free paper) Notes: Includes bibliographical references (p. [178]-189) and index. Subjects: AIDS (Disease)--Africa. LC Classification: RA644.A25 B35 1992b Dewey Class No.: 362.1/969792/0096 20

Barnett, Tony. AIDS in Africa: its present and future impact / Tony Barnett and Piers Blaikie. Published/Created: London: Belhaven Press, 1992. Related Authors: Blaikie, Piers M. Description: ix, 193 p.: ill.; 24 cm. ISBN: 1852931159: Notes: Includes bibliographical references (p. [178]-189) and index. Subjects: AIDS (Disease)--Africa. LC Classification: RA644.A25 B35 1992 Dewey Class No.: 362.1/969792/0096 20

Bongaarts, John, 1945- Modeling the spread of HIV and the demographic impact of AIDS in Africa / John Bongaarts. Published/Created: New York,

N.Y. (1 Dag Hammarskjold Plaza, New York 10017): Population Council, [1988]. Description: 42 p.: ill.; 23 cm. Notes: Cover title. Includes bibliographical references (p. 38-40) Subjects: AIDS (Disease)--Epidemiology--Computer simulation. AIDS (Disease)--Africa--Epidemiology--Computer simulation. Series: Working papers (Population Council. Center for Policy Studies); no. 140. Variant Series: Working papers / Center for Policy Studies; no. 140 (Oct. 1988) LC Classification: RA644.A25 B66 1988 Dewey Class No.: 614.5/993 20

Broomberg, Jonathan. The economic impact of the AIDS epidemic in South Africa / Jonathan Broomberg, Patrick Masobe, Malcolm Steinberg. Published/Created: Cape Town: Economic Trends Research Group, Development Policy Research Unit, University of Cape Town, 1991. Related Authors: Masobe, Patrick. Steinberg, Malcolm (Malcolm H.) Description: 60 p.; 21 cm. Notes: Includes bibliographical references (p. 58-60). Subjects: AIDS (Disease)--Economic aspects--South Africa. AIDS (Disease)--South Africa--Epidemiology. Series: Working papers (Economic Trends Research Group (Cape Town, South Africa); no. 5. Variant Series: ET working paper; no. 5 LC Classification: RA644.A25 B753 1991 Dewey Class No.: 362.1969792/00968 21

Campbell, Catherine. Managing HIV/AIDS in South Africa: lessons from industrial settings / Catherine Campbell, Brian Williams and Catherine MacPhail. Published/Created: Auckland Park: CSIR, 1999. ISBN: 0798854340

Chirimuuta, Richard C. (Richard Chidau) AIDS, Africa, and racism / Richard C. Chirimuuta, Rosalind J. Chirimuuta. Edition Information: New and rev. ed. Published/Created: London: Free Association Books, 1989. Related Authors: Chirimuuta, Rosalind J. (Rosalind Joan). Description: 192 p.; 22 cm. ISBN: 1853430722 Notes: Includes bibliographical references and index. Subjects: AIDS (Disease)--Africa. AIDS (Disease)--Etiology. AIDS (Disease)--Public opinion. LC Classification: RA644.A25 C45 1989 Dewey Class No.: 362.1/969792/0096 20

Chirimuuta, Richard C. (Richard Chidau) Aids, Africa, and racism / Richard C. Chirimuuta,

Rosalind J. Chirimuuta.
Published/Created: [Stanhope,
Bretby, Nr Burton-on-Trent,
Derbyshire, U.K.]: R.C.
Chirimuuta, 1987. Related
Authors: Chirimuuta, Rosalind
J. (Rosalind Joan). Description:
160 p.; 22 cm. ISBN:
0951280414 (pbk.):
0951280406 (hard) Notes: Title
on half t.p.: Aids, Africa &
racism. Includes bibliographical
references. Subjects: AIDS
(Disease)--Africa. AIDS
(Disease)--Etiology. AIDS
(Disease)--Public opinion. LC
Classification: RA644.A25
C45x 1987

Critical choices for the NGO
   community: African
   development in the 1990s.
   Published/Created: [Edinburgh:
   University of Edinburgh, Centre
   of African Studies, 1990]
   Related Authors: University of
   Edinburgh. Centre of African
   Studies. SCIAF. Description:
   302 p.; 21 cm. Contents:
   Conference themes: an
   interpretative summary /
   Christopher Fyfe -- African
   NGO decolonisation: a critical
   choice for the 1990s / Kingston
   Kajese -- Northern NGOs in
   Southern Africa: some heretical
   thoughts / Robin Palmer &
   Jenny Rossiter -- Judging
   success: evaluating NGO
   approaches to alleviating

poverty in developing countries
/ Roger Riddell -- Alternative
financing strategies for NGOs /
Fernand Vincent, Piers
Campbell -- NGO-donor
government relations: new
challenges, new potential / Guy
Mustard -- Government-NGO
relationship in the context of
alternative development
strategies in Africa / Njuguna
Ng'ethe, Winnie Mitullah,
Mutahi Ngunyi -- Governments
and NGOs: an unacknowledged
conspiracy? / Achmat Dangor --
Monitoring human rights in
Africa: a contribution to
development? / Louise Pirouet -
- Increasing frequency of
disaster relief in Africa: what
has gone wrong? / Sithembiso
Nyoni -- Disabled people in
development: challenging
traditional attitudes / Chris
Underhill -- NGOs and
government: their role in
community self-empowerment
and the case of HIV and AIDS /
Steve McGarry -- African
NGOs: do they have a future? /
Odhiambo Anacleti -- NGO's,
politics and the state: parallels
and parting thoughts / Chris
Allen. Notes: On cover: SCIAF.
"Proceedings of a conference
held in the Centre of African
Studies, University of
Edinburgh, 24 & 25 May 1990".
Text on lining papers. Includes
bibliographies. Subjects: Non-

governmental organizations--
Congresses. Africa--Economic
conditions--Congresses. Africa--
Economic policy--Congresses.
Organisations Africa Series:
Seminar proceedings
(University of Edinburgh.
Centre of African Studies); no
30. Variant Series: Seminar
proceedings; no 30 LC
Classification: ACQUISITION
IN PROCESS (COPIED)
(lccopycat) National Bib. No.:
GB91-19777

Declaration on the AIDS Epidemic
in Africa, July 1992 =
Déclaration sur l'épidemie de
SIDA en Afrique, juillet 1992 =
Declaração sobre a Epidemia de
SIDA em Africa, julho 1992 =
Al-A`l¯an al-Kh¯as Bawb¯a' al-
AYDIZ f¯i Ifr¯iqi¯a Tamawz,
Y¯uly¯u 1992.
Published/Created: [Addis
Ababa]: Organization of African
Unity, [1992] Related Authors:
Organization of African Unity.
Description: 17 p.; 30 cm.
Notes: Arabic, English, French,
and Portuguese. Subjects:
Organization of African Unity--
Positions. AIDS (Disease)--
Africa. LC Classification:
RA643.86.A35 D43 1992

East Africa AIDS NGOS
Networking Workshop (1994:
MS-TCDC) Networking: "a
strategy for strengthening AIDS

NGOs programs in East Africa":
workshop proceedings / report
by Organising Committee
Published/Created: Arusha,
Tanzania: AIDS NGOS
Network East Africa, [1994?]
Related Authors: East Africa
AIDS NGOS Networking
Workshop (1994: MS-TCDC).
Organising Committee.
Description: 99 p.: ill.; 30 cm.
Notes: "26th-29th September,
1994, MS-TCDC, Usa River
Arusha, Tanzania." "East Africa
AIDS NGOS Networking
Workshop"--P. 70. LC
Classification: IN PROCESS

East African Literature Bureau.
Catalogue of books and visual
aids published by or in
association with East African
Literature Bureau and available
from bookshops throughout East
Africa. Published/Created:
Kampala. Description: v. 22
cm. Current Frequency: Annual
Subjects: Text-books--Africa,
East--Bibliography--
Catalogs.Visual aids--Catalogs.
LC Classification: Z5819 .E15

Eskom Conference & Exhibition
Centre. AIDS and your
response: proceedings, 11-14
November 1992, Eskom
Conference & Exhibition
Centre, Midrand, South Africa /
organized by the Institute of
World Concerns (IWC), in

conjunction with the Churches AIDS Programme (CAP), and the University of South Africa (UNISA), with the assistance of conference planners. Published/Created: Halfway House, Republic of South Africa: Institute of World Concerns, c1992. Related Authors: Institute of World Concerns. Methodist Church of Southern Africa. Churches AIDS Programme. University of South Africa. Description: 1 v. (various pagings): ill.; 21 cm. ISBN: 062017319X Notes: Includes bibliographical references and index. Subjects: AIDS (Disease)--Africa--Congresses. LC Classification: RA644.A25 E83 1992 Dewey Class No.: 362.1/969792/00968 20

Facing up to AIDS: the socio-economic impact in Southern Africa / edited by Sholto Cross and Alan Whiteside. Published/Created: New York: St. Martin's Press, 1993. Related Authors: Cross, Sholto. Whiteside, Alan. Description: xi, 331 p.: ill.; 23 cm. ISBN: 0312091060 Notes: Includes bibliographical references and index. Subjects: AIDS (Disease)--Africa, Southern--Social aspects. AIDS (Disease)--Africa, Southern--Economic aspects. LC Classification:

RA644.A25 F33 1993 Dewey Class No.: 362.1/9697/9200968 20

Frontline. Born in Africa: a Frontline AIDS Quarterly special edition. Published/Created: United States: WETA-TV, 1990-04-03. Related Authors: WETA-TV (Television station: Washington, D.C.) LC Off-Air Taping Collection (Library of Congress) Description: 2 videocassettes of 2 (ca. 90 min.): sd., col.; 3/4 in. viewing copy. Notes: Copyright: reg. unknown. No. 809. Time of broadcast: Tuesday, 9 PM-10:30 PM. Source of Acquisition: Received: 7/2/90 from LC video lab; viewing copy; off-air taping, LWO 24998; LC Off-Air Taping Collection. Genre/Form: Television. Series. Video. LC Classification: VBG 7035-7036 (viewing copy)

Global health: U.S. agency for international development fights AIDS in Africa, but better data needed to measure impact: report to the Chairman, Subcommittee on African Affairs, Committee on Foreign Relations, U.S. Senate / United States General Accounting Office. Published/Created: Washington, D.C.: The Office, [2001] Related Authors: United States. General Accounting

Office. Description: 48 p.: ill., maps; 28 cm. Notes: Cover title. "March 2001." "GAO-01-449."

Green, Edward C. (Edward Crocker), 1944- AIDS and STDs in Africa: bridging the gap between traditional healing and modern medicine / Edward C. Green. Published/Created: Boulder, Colo.: Westview Press, 1994. Description: xi, 276 p.: ill.; 23 cm. ISBN: 0813378478 Notes: Includes bibliographical references (p. 251-265) and index. Subjects: Sexually transmitted diseases--Africa. AIDS (Disease)--Africa. Traditional medicine--Africa. LC Classification: RA644.V4 G74 1994 Dewey Class No.: 362.1/96951/0096 20

Grose, Robert Nicholas. AIDS: proposals for action: the global epidemic and the crisis in Africa / prepared by Robert Grose for War on Want. Published/Created: London: War on Want, 1987. Related Authors: War on Want (Organization) Description: iii, 47, [4], 5 p.; 30 cm. Notes: Cover title. "May 1987." Includes bibliographical references (p. 45-47). Subjects: AIDS (Disease)--Africa. AIDS (Disease)--Africa--Transmission. LC

Classification: RA644.A25 G762 1987 Dewey Class No.: 362.1/969792/0096 20

Histories of sexually transmitted diseases and HIV/AIDS in Sub-Saharan Africa / edited by Philip W. Setel, Milton Lewis, and Maryinez Lyons. Published/Created: Westport, Conn.: Greenwood Press, 1999. Related Authors: Setel, Philip. Lewis, Milton James. Lyons, Maryinez. Description: 267 p.: ill.; 24 cm. ISBN: 0313297150 (alk. paper) Notes: "Selected bibliography": p. [245]-254. Includes bibliographical references and index. Subjects: Sexually transmitted diseases--Africa, Sub-Saharan History. AIDS (Disease)--Africa-Sub-Saharan--History. Series: Contributions in medical studies, 0886-8220; no. 44 LC Classification: RA644.V4 H55 1999 Dewey Class No.: 616.95/1/00967 21

HIV prevention and AIDS care in Africa: a district level approach / Japheth Ng'weshemi ... [et al.], editors. Published/Created: Amsterdam: Royal Tropical Institute, c1997. Related Authors: Ng'weshemi, Japheth. Description: 400 p.: ill.; 24 cm. ISBN: 9068321080 Notes: Includes bibliographical references. Subjects: HIV infections--Africa. AIDS (Disease)--Africa. HIV Infections--prevention & control--Africa. Acquired Immunodeficiency Syndrome. Community Health Services--Africa. LC Classification: RA644.A25 H5935 1997 Dewey Class No.: 362.1/969792/0096 21

HIV/AIDS in Africa.
Published/Created: Washington, D.C.: Health Studies Branch, International Programs Center, Population Division, U.S. Bureau of the Census, 1995. Related Authors: International Programs Center (U.S.). Health Studies Branch. International Conference on AIDS and STDs in Africa (9th: 1995: Kampala, Uganda) Description: 1 v. (various pagings): ill.; 28 cm. Notes: "Prepared for the IX International Conference on AIDS and STDs in Africa, Kampala, Uganda, December 10-14, 1995." Includes bibliographical references. Subjects: AIDS (Disease)--Africa--Congresses. HIV infections--Africa--Congresses. Series: Research note (International Programs Center (U.S.). Health Studies Branch); no. 20. Variant Series: Research note; no. 20 LC Classification: RA644.A25 .H57547 1995

Dewey Class No.: 614.5/993 20

Implications of AIDS for demography and policy in Southern Africa / edited by Alan Whiteside. Published/Created: Pietermaritzburg: University of Natal Press, 1998. Related Authors: Whiteside, Alan. Description: 146 p.: ill.; 24 cm. ISBN: 0869809407 Notes: Includes bibliographical references.

Intensifying action against HIV/AIDS in Africa: responding to a development crisis. Published/Created: Washington, DC: World Bank, Africa Region, c2000. Related Authors: World Bank. Africa Regional Office. Description: xi, 89, [1] p.: ill., 1 col. map; 24 cm. ISBN: 0821345729 Notes: "World Bank 2000"--Cover. Includes bibliographical references. Subjects: AIDS (Disease)--Africa. LC Classification: RA644.A25 I573 2000 Dewey Class No.: 362.1/969792/0096 21

International Conference on AIDS and Associated Cancers in Africa (3rd: 1988: Arusha, Tanzania) Third International Conference on AIDS and Associated Cancers in Africa: final programme: September 14-16, 1988, Arusha International

Conference Centre, Arusha,
Tanzania / sponsored by the
Medical Association of
Tanzania ... [et al.].
Published/Created: [Dar es
Salaam]: The Association,
[1988- Related Authors:
Medical Association of
Tanzania. Description: v.: ill.;
30 cm. Notes: Cover AIDS and
associated cancers in Africa.
Holdings listed alphabetically
by volume title. LC has:
Abstracts volume; Final
programme. Subjects: AIDS
(Disease)--Congresses. AIDS
(Disease)--Africa--Congresses.
LC Classification: RC607.A26
I57 1988 Dewey Class No.:
616.97/92 20

International Conference on AIDS in
Africa (8th: 1992: Yaounde,
Cameroon) VIIe Conférence
internationale sur le SIDA en
Afrique: 08-11 Décembre 1992,
Yaoundé, Cameroun = VIIth
International Conference on
AIDS in Africa: December 08-
11, 1992. Published/Created:
[Yaoundé, Cameroun]:
Challenge Graphics Vision,
[1992] Description: 2 v.; 30
cm. Contents: [Vol. 1].
Programme final et livre des
résumés -- [v. 2]. Call for
abstract, last announcement.
Notes: Cover title. English and
French. Subjects: AIDS
(Disease)--Africa--Congresses.

LC Classification: RA644.A35
I68 1992 Dewey Class No.:
616.97/92/0096 20

Jackson, Helen. AIDS home care: a
baseline survey in Zimbabwe /
[researched and compiled by
Helen Jackson, Kate Mhambi;
editor, Viola Zimunya].
Published/Created: Kopje,
Harare, Zimbabwe: Journal of
social development in Africa,
School of Social Work, c1992.
Related Authors: Mhambi, Kate.
Zimunya, Viola. Description:
48 p.: ill.; 30 cm. ISBN:
0797411437 Notes: Includes
bibliographical references (p.
37-38). Subjects: AIDS
(Disease)--Patients--Home care-
-Zimbabwe. Series: Research
series (School of Social Work
(Harare, Zimbabwe). Research
Unit); no. 3. Variant Series:
Research series / Research Unit,
School of Social Work; no. 3
LC Classification: RA644.A25
J293 1992 Dewey Class No.:
362.1/969792/0096891 20

Jackson, Helen. Family coping and
AIDS in Zimbabwe: a study /
[researched and compiled by
Helen Jackson, assisted by Kate
Mhambi; edited by Nigel Hall].
Published/Created: Harare:
Journal of social development in
Africa, School of Social Work,
c1994. Related Authors:
Mhambi, Kate. Hall, Nigel.

Description: 72 p.: ill.; 30 cm. ISBN: 079741357X Notes: Includes bibliographical references (p. 39-40). Subjects: AIDS (Disease)--Patients--Zimbabwe--Family relationships. AIDS (Disease)--Zimbabwe. Series: Research series (School of Social Work (Harare, Zimbabwe). Research Unit); no. 4. Variant Series: Research Unit series / Research Unit, School of Social Work; no. 4 LC Classification: RC607.A26 J323 1994 Dewey Class No.: 362.1/969792/0096891 21

Lamboray, Jean-Louis, 1947-
Combatting AIDS and the other sexually transmitted diseases in Africa: a review of the World Bank's agenda for action / Jean-Louis Lamboray, A. Edward Elmendorf. Published/Created: Washington, D.C.: World Bank, c1992. Related Authors: Elmendorf, A. Edward, 1938-World Bank. Description: xii, 34 p.: ill.; 28 cm. ISBN: 0821322621 Notes: Includes bibliographical references (p. 33-34). Subjects: AIDS (Disease)--Africa. Sexually transmitted diseases--Africa. Acquired Immunodeficiency Syndrome--prevention & control Africa. Sexually Transmitted Diseases--prevention & control Africa.

Series: World Bank discussion papers; 181. World Bank discussion papers. Africa Technical Department series. Variant Series: World Bank discussion papers, 0259-210X; 181. Africa Technical Department series LC Classification: RA644.A25 L35 1992 Dewey Class No.: 362.1/9697/920096 20

List of lights, radio aids, and fog signals. The west coasts of Europe and Africa, the Mediterranean Sea, Black Sea, and Azovskoye More (Sea of Azov) / prepared and published by the Defense Mapping Agency Hydrographic/Topographic Center. Portion of West coasts of Europe and Africa, the Mediterranean Sea, Black Sea, and Azovskoye More (Sea of Azov) Spine Lights. West coast of Europe Published/Created: Bethesda, MD: The Center: For sale by authorized sales agents of the National Ocean Service, Related Authors: United States. Defense Mapping Agency. Hydrographic/Topographic Center. United States. National Imagery and Mapping Agency. Description: v.: ill.; 26-28 cm. Current Frequency: Annual Separated from: United States. Defense Mapping Agency. Hydrographic/Topographic

Center. List of lights and fog signals 0096-1280 (DLC) 80647739 (OCoLC)6767321 Cancel/Invalid LCCN: sn 94028075 Notes: Description based on: 1994; title from cover. Vols. for 19 -1996 prepared and published by: the Defense Mapping Agency Hydrographic/Topographic Center; 1997- by: the National Imagery and Mapping Agency. SERBIB/SERLOC merged record Kept up-to-date between eds. by: Notice to mariners. Notice to mariners 0092-1262 (DLC) 80640564 (OCoLC)4507973 Subjects: Aids to navigation--Atlantic Coast (Europe)--Lists. Aids to navigation--Atlantic Coast (Africa)--Lists. Aids to navigation--Mediterranean Sea--Lists. Aids to navigation--Black Sea--Lists. Aids to navigation--Azov, Sea of (Ukraine and Russia) Lists. Series: Pub. (United States. Defense Mapping Agency. Hydrographic/Topographic Center); 113. Pub. (United States. National Imagery and Mapping Agency); 113. Variant Series: Pub.; 113 LC Classification: VK1151 .L565 Dewey Class No.: 387.1/55/094 20 Govt. Doc. No.: D 5.317:113/ D 5.317/2:113

Loewenson, Rene. Social and economic issues of HIV/AIDS in southern Africa / by Rene Loewenson and Alan Whiteside. Published/Created: Avondale, Harare, Zimbabwe: Southern Africa AIDS Information Dissemination Service, [1997] Related Authors: Whiteside, Alan. Southern Africa AIDS Information Dissemination Service. Description: vii, 104 p.: ill.; 30 cm. ISBN: 0797417338 Notes: "March 1997." "A consultancy report prepared for SAFAIDS, Harare." Includes bibliographical references (p. 90-104). Subjects: AIDS (Disease)--Economic aspects--Africa, Southern. AIDS (Disease)--Social aspects--Africa, Southern. Series: SAfAIDS occasional paper series; no. 2 LC Classification: RA643.86.A356 L64 1997 Dewey Class No.: 362.1/969792/00968 21

Maclean, Gordon L. Aids to bird identification in southern Africa / Gordon L. Maclean; illustrated by Linda Davis. Edition Information: 2nd ed. Published/Created: Pietermaritzburg: University of Natal Press, 1987 (1988 printing) Description: x, 61, [2] p.: ill.; 21 cm. ISBN: 086980586X Notes: Includes bibliographical references (p. [62]-[63]). Subjects: Birds--Africa, Southern--Identification. LC Classification: QL692.A435 M33 1987

Maclean, Gordon L. Aids to bird identification in Southern Africa / Gordon L. Maclean; illustrated by Linda Davis. Published/Created: Pietermaritzburg: University of Natal Press, 1981. Description: ix, 54 p.: ill.; 21 cm. ISBN: 0869802615 LC Classification: MLCS 82/9759

Mati, J. K. G. AIDS, women, and children in Africa: (the impact of AIDS on reproductive health) / J.K.G. Mati. Published/Created: Nairobi, Kenya: IRHTR Occasional Publications, c1997. Related Authors: Consultative Meeting on AIDS and Reproductive Health in Africa (1st: 1987: Mombasa, Kenya) Consultative Meeting on AIDS and Reproductive Health in Africa (2nd: 1991: Mombasa, Kenya) Description: xiv, 180 p.: ill. (1 col.), map; 21 cm. Cancelled ISBN: 996699580 Notes: "... Consultative Meeting on AIDS and Reproductive Health in Africa ..."--Pref. Includes bibliographical references and index. Subjects: AIDS (Disease)--Africa. AIDS

(Disease) in women--Africa. AIDS (Disease) in children--Africa. LC Classification: RA644.A25 M384 1997 Dewey Class No.: 362.1/969792/0096 21

Mezerik, A. G. (Avrahm G.), 1901-ed. Economic development aids for underdeveloped countries: UN sources, national and int'l agencies, financial and technical assistance [with] special section on Africa. Published/Created: [New York, International Review Service, 1961] Description: 108 p. illus. 28 cm. Subjects: Economic assistance. Developing countries. Series: International review service, v. 7, no. 63 LC Classification: D839.3 .I56 vol. 7, no. 63 Dewey Class No.: 338.91

Mupedziswa, Rodreck. AIDS in Africa: the social work response / Rodreck Mupedziswa. Running Social work response Published/Created: Harare: Journal of social development in Africa, School of Social Work, c1998. Description: xxi, 153 p.: ill.; 21 cm. ISBN: 0797419373 Notes: Includes bibliographical references (p. 145-152). Subjects: Medical social work--Africa. AIDS (Disease)--Patients--Services for--Africa. AIDS (Disease)--Patients--Home care--Africa. LC

Classification: HV687.5.A35 M86 1998

Mwale, Genevieve. Women and AIDS in rural Africa: rural womens' views of AIDS in Zambia / Genevieve Mwale, Philip Burnard. Published/Created: Aldershot; Brookfield, USA: Avebury, c1992. Related Authors: Burnard, Philip. Description: viii, 127 p.; 23 cm. ISBN: 1856283968 Notes: Includes bibliographical references (p. 106-122) and index. Subjects: AIDS (Disease) in women--Zambia. Women--Zambia--Attitudes. Acquired Immunodeficiency Syndrome. Health Surveys--Zambia. Rural Health--Zambia. Women's Health. LC Classification: RA644.A25 M9 1992 Dewey Class No.: 362.1/997/920096894 20

Napolitano, Gaetano. L'emploi des audio-visuels en Afrique; contribution du CIDAECA au Colloque Image et son, Alger, 26 avril-3 mai 1965. Audio-visual aids in Africa; contribution of CIDAECA at the "Image et son" Meeting, Algiers, April 26th-May 3rd, 1965. Published/Created: Como, P. Cairoli [1966] Related Authors: Cepollaro, Armando. Bartocci, Enzo.

International Committee for the Development of Educational and Cultural Activities in Africa. "Image et son" Meeting (1965: Algiers) Description: 62 p. 25 cm. Contents: Suggestions pour le progrès accéléré des masses africaines, par G. Napolitano.--Suggestions for a faster progress of African masses, by G. Napolitano.--Avant-projet d'une coopération inter-africaine pour la production et la circulation des matériaux audio-visuels au service de l'éducation et de l'information, par A. Cepollaro.--Draft-plan on an inter-African co-operation for producing and distributing audio-visual material in the service of education and information, by A. Cepollaro.--Le rôle de l'énergie dans l'enseignement et l'information, par E. Bartocci.--The role of electric power in teaching and information, by E. Bartocci. Notes: At head of Napolitano. Cepollaro. Bartocci. Includes bibliographical references. Subjects: Audio-visual education--Africa. Series: Quaderni d'Africa; n. 2. Variant Series: Pubblicazioni dell'Istituto italiano per l'Africa. Serie 1: Quaderni d'Africa, n. 2 LC Classification: LB1043 .N26

National Association of Child Care Workers (South Africa).

Conference (9th: 1993: Johannesburg, South Africa) Children and youth at risk: HIV/AIDS issues, residential care, and community perspectives: presentations from the first all-Africa conference and ninth biennial Conference of the National Association of Child Care Workers / edited by Brian Gannon. Published/Created: Cape Town: NACCW, 1994. Related Authors: Gannon, Brian. Description: 162 p.; 21 cm. ISBN: 0958394911 Notes: Includes bibliographical references. Subjects: Children--Institutional care--Africa--Congresses. Problem children--Institutional care--Africa--Congresses. Social work with children--Africa--Congresses. AIDS (Disease) in children--South Africa--Congresses. LC Classification: HV866.A35 N37 1994

National Research Council (U.S.). Panel on Data and Research Priorities for Arresting AIDS in Sub-Saharan Africa. Preventing and mitigating AIDS in Sub-Saharan Africa: research and data priorities for the social and behavioral sciences / Barney Cohen and James Trussell, editors; Panel on Data and Research Priorities for Arresting AIDS in Sub-Saharan Africa, Committee on Population, Commission on Behavioral and Social Sciences and Education, National Research Council. Published/Created: Washington, D.C.: National Academy Press, 1996. Related Authors: Cohen, Barney, 1959- Trussell, James. Description: xi, 356 p.: ill., maps; 23 cm. ISBN: 030905480X Notes: Includes bibliographical references (p. 271-314) and index. Subjects: AIDS (Disease)--Africa, Sub-Saharan. LC Classification: RA644.A25 N264 1996 Dewey Class No.: 614.5/993 20

Network of AIDS Researchers of Eastern and Southern Africa. Membership directory / Network of AIDS Researchers of Eastern and Southern Africa (NARESA). Published/Created: Nairobi, Kenya: NARESA, [1992- Description: v.; 21 cm. 1992- Current Frequency: Annual Notes: Title from cover. SERBIB/SERLOC merged record Subjects: AIDS (Disease)--Research--Africa, Eastern--Directories Periodicals. AIDS (Disease)--Research--Africa, Southern--Directories Periodicals. LC Classification: RA858.A1 N47 Dewey Class No.: 616.97/92/00720676 20

Network of AIDS Researchers of Eastern and Southern Africa.

Newsletter / Network of AIDS Researchers of Eastern and Southern Africa. Published/Created: Nairobi, Kenya: NARESA, [1989- Description: v.: ill.; 30 cm. No. 1 (May 1989)- Current Frequency: Quarterly, June 1992- Former Frequency: Annual, May 1989-June 1991 Notes: Title from caption. SERBIB/SERLOC merged record Subjects: Network of AIDS Researchers of Eastern and Southern Africa. AIDS (Disease)--Africa, Eastern--Periodicals. AIDS (Disease)--Africa, Southern--Periodicals. Acquired Immunodeficiency Syndrome--prevention & control Africa, Southern--periodicals. HIV Infections--prevention & control--Africa, Southern periodicals. LC Classification: RA644.A25 N4724a Dewey Class No.: 616.97/92/0096 20

Network of AIDS Researchers of Eastern and Southern Africa. Report of activities / Network of AIDS Researchers of Eastern and Southern Africa. Published/Created: Nairobi, Kenya: NARESA, Description: v.; 30 cm. Current Frequency: Annual Notes: Description based on: 1992; title from cover. SERBIB/SERLOC merged record Subjects: AIDS

(Disease)--Africa, Eastern--Periodicals. AIDS (Disease)--Africa, Southern--Periodicals. LC Classification: RA644.A25 N47243a Dewey Class No.: 362.1/969792/0096 20

Packard, Randall M., 1945- Epidemiologists, social scientists, and the structure of medical research on AIDS in Africa / by Randall M. Packard. Published/Created: Boston, MA (270 Bay State Rd., Boston 02215): African Studies Center, Boston University, 1989. Description: 19 leaves: ill.; 28 cm. Notes: Includes bibliographical references. Subjects: AIDS (Disease)--Africa--Epidemiology--Research. Series: Working papers in African studies (Boston, Mass.); no. 137. Variant Series: Working papers in African studies; no. 137 LC Classification: RA644.A25 P33 1989 Dewey Class No.: 614.5/993 20

Presidential Mission on Children Orphaned by AIDS in Sub-Saharan Africa (U.S.) Report on the presidential mission on children orphaned by AIDS in Sub-Saharan Africa: findings and plan of action. Published/Created: Washington, D.C. (736 Jackson Place, Washington 20503): Office of

National AIDS Policy, [1999] Related Authors: United States. Office of National AIDS Policy. Description: 36 p.: ill.; 28 cm. Notes: Cover title. "The White House, July 19, 1999"--Cover. Shipping list no.: 99-0373-P. Includes bibliographical references (p. 35). Additional Form Avail.: Also available via Internet from the ONAP web site (PDF file only). Address as of 10-19-99: http://www.whitehouse.gov/ONAP/pub/africa2.pdf; curent access is available via PURL. Subjects: AIDS (Disease)--Africa, Sub-Saharan. Orphans--Africa, Sub-Saharan. Children--Africa, Sub-Saharan. Govt. Doc. No.: PREX 1.2:OR 7

Provincial population projections, 1996-2021. High HIV/Aids impact / compiled by JM Calitz. Published/Created: Halfway House: Development Bank of Southern Africa, [2000] Related Authors: Calitz, J. M. Description: vi, 144 p.: ill.; 21x30 cm. ISBN: 191969255X Notes: "September 2000." Subjects: Population forecasting--South Africa--Statistics. HIV infections--South Africa--Statistics. Life expectancy--South Africa--Statistics. South Africa--Population--Statistics. Series: Development paper

(Development Bank of Southern Africa); 144. Variant Series: Development paper; 144 LC Classification: HA4701 .P765 2000

Provincial population projections, 1996-2021. Low HIV/Aids impact / JM Calitz, comp. Published/Created: Halfway House: Development Bank of Southern Africa, [2000] Related Authors: Calitz, J. M. Description: viii, 144 p.: ill.; 21x29 cm. ISBN: 1919692541 Notes: "August 2000." Subjects: Population forecasting--South Africa--Statistics. HIV infections--South Africa--Statistics. Life expectancy--South Africa--Statistics. South Africa--Population--Statistics. Series: Development paper (Development Bank of Southern Africa); 143. Variant Series: Development paper; 143 LC Classification: HA4701 .P766 1999

Regional Consultative Meeting on AIDS Research Needs in Africa (1987: Mombasa, Kenya) AIDS and reproductive health in Africa: a report of a Regional Consultative Meeting on AIDS Research Needs in Africa, Mombasa, Kenya, 9th to 13th November 1987. Published/Created: Nairobi,

Kenya: African Fertility Society, c1988. Related Authors: African Fertility Society. Description: ix, 42 p.; 22 cm. Subjects: AIDS (Disease)--Africa--Congresses. LC Classification: RA644.A25 R45 1987 Dewey Class No.: 362.1/969792/0096 20

Saayman, W. A. (Willem A.) AIDS, the leprosy of our time?: towards a Christian response to AIDS in southern and central Africa / Willem Saayman, Jacques Kriel. Edition Information: 1st ed. Published/Created: Johannesburg: Orion, 1992. Related Authors: Kriel, J. R. Description: 83 p.; 19 cm. ISBN: 0798706058 Notes: Includes bibliographical references (p. 80-83). Subjects: AIDS (Disease)--Religious aspects--Christianity. AIDS (Disease)--Africa. AIDS (Disease)--Social aspects--Africa. LC Classification: BV4460.7 .S22 1992 Dewey Class No.: 261.8/321969792 20

Sadie, Y. (Yolande) AIDS in Africa and its impact on the South African mining industry / Y. Sadie, M. van Aardt, A. von Below. Published/Created: [Pretoria]: Africa Institute of South Africa, 1993. Related Authors: Van Aardt, M. (Maxie)

Von Below, A. (Anton) Description: 10 leaves; 30 cm. ISBN: 0798301120 Notes: Includes bibliographical references (leaves 9-10). Subjects: Miners--Health and hygiene--South Africa. Mineral industries--Employees--Health and hygiene--South Africa. Migrant labor--Health and hygiene--South Africa. Alien labor--Health and hygiene--South Africa. Miners--Medical examinations--South Africa. HIV infections--South Africa. AIDS (Disease)--South Africa. Mineral industries--Labor productivity--South Africa. Series: Occasional papers of the Africa Institute; no. 56. Variant Series: Africa Institute occasional paper; no. 56 LC Classification: HD7269.M61 S67 1993

Sai, Fred T. Why is Africa losing the battle against AIDS? / Fred T. Sai. Published/Created: Accra: Ghana Academy of Arts & Sciences, [1999] Description: 24 p.; 20 cm. Notes: Cover title. "November 1999." Includes bibliographical references (p. 24). LC Classification: MLCS 2000/00885 (H)

Schlettwein, Carl. Libraries and archives in South West Africa / C. Schlettwein and L. Gebhardt.

Bibliographical aids for studies on South West Africa / M. Vogt. Towards standards of accuracy and reliability in the bibliography of Ghana language materials / H. M. J. Trutenau. Published/Created: Basel: Basler Afrika Bibliographien, 1975. Related Authors: Gebhardt, Lisa, joint author. Vogt, Martin. Bibliographical aids for studies on South West Africa. 1975. Trutenau, H. M. J. (H. Max J.). Towards standards of accuracy and reliability in the bibliography of Ghana language materials. 1975. Description: 56 p.; 21 cm. Subjects: Libraries--Namibia. Archives--Namibia. Namibia--Bibliography of bibliographies. Ghana--Imprints--Bibliography--Methodology. Series: Mitteilungen der Basler Afrika Bibliographien; v. 13. Variant Series: Communications from the Basel Africa Bibliography; v. 13 LC Classification: Z857.S77 S34 Dewey Class No.: 021/.00968

Schmidt, Nancy J. Resources for teaching about the social impact of AIDS in Africa / Nancy J. Schmidt. Published/Created: Bloomington, IN: African Studies Program, Indiana University, [1990] Description: 24 p.; 28 cm. Notes: Cover title. "January 1990." Subjects:

AIDS (Disease)--Social aspects--Africa--Study and teaching. AIDS (Disease)--Social aspects--Africa--Bibliography. LC Classification: RA644.A25 S35 1990 Dewey Class No.: 362.1/969792/0096 20

Shorter, Aylward. The church and AIDS in Africa: a case study: Nairobi City / by Aylward Shorter & Edwin Onyancha. Published/Created: Nairobi, Kenya: Paulines Publications Africa, 1998. Related Authors: Onyancha, Edwin. Description: 141 p.; 21 cm. Cancelled ISBN: 996621384X Notes: Includes bibliographical references. LC Classification: IN PROCESS

Small, Alison. The effects of HIV/AIDS on farming systems in Eastern Africa / [producer], FAO Farm Management and Production Economics Service. Published/Created: Rome: Food and Agriculture Organization of the United Nations, 1995. Related Authors: Barnett, Tony. Haslwimmer, Martina. Food and Agriculture Organization of the United Nations. Farm Management and Production Economics Service. Description: xi, 173 p.: ill., maps; 21 cm. ISBN: 925103611X Notes: "Based on the contributions of two main authors ... Tony Barnett ... [and]

Martina Haslwimmer"--P. iii. "Alison Small was in charge of drafting and editing the text"--P. iv. Includes bibliographical references (p. 171-173). Subjects: Agricultural systems--Africa, Eastern. HIV (Viruses)--Africa, Eastern. AIDS (Disease)--Africa, Eastern. Africa, Eastern--Rural conditions. LC Classification: S472.A354 S535 1995

The Continuing HIV/AIDS epidemic in Africa: responses and coping strategies / edited by I.O. Orubuloye, John C. Caldwell and James P.M. Ntozi. Published/Created: Canberra: Health Transition Centre, National Centre for Epidemiology and Population Health, Australian National University, 1999 . Related Authors: Ntozi, James P. M. Caldwell, John C. (John Charles), 1928- Orubuloye, I. O. (Israel Olatunji), 1947- Australian National University. Health Transition Centre. Description: 236 p.; 25 cm. Notes: Bibliography: p. 234-236. Subjects: AIDS (Disease)--Africa. Acquired immunodeficiency syndrome.

The Handbook for AIDS prevention in Africa / editors, Peter Lamptey, Peter Piot; with the assistance of Robert Gringle.

Published/Created: Durham, N.C., USA: Family Health International, 1990- Related Authors: Lamptey, Peter Richter. Piot, Peter, 1949- Gringle, Robert. Family Health International (Organization) Description: 1 v. (loose-leaf): ill.; maps; 30 cm. ISBN: 0939704064 Notes: Includes bibliographical references. Subjects: AIDS (Disease)--Africa--Prevention. AIDS (Disease)--Africa--Epidemiology. Acquired Immunodeficiency Syndrome--epidemiology--Africa. Acquired Immunodeficiency Syndrome--prevention & control Africa. LC Classification: RA644.A25 H36 1990 Dewey Class No.: 614.5/993 20

The Heterosexual transmission of AIDS in Africa / edited by Dieter Koch-Weser and Hannelore Vanderschmidt. Published/Created: Cambridge, Mass.: Abt Books, c1988. Related Authors: Koch-Weser, Dieter K. Vanderschmidt, Hannelore F. Description: xv, 293 p.: ill.; 28 cm. ISBN: 0890116040 (pbk.: alk. paper): 0890116032 (hard: alk. paper) Notes: Includes bibliographies and indexes. Subjects: AIDS (Disease)--Transmission--Africa. AIDS (Disease)--Africa--Epidemiology. Heterosexuals--

Health and hygiene. LC Classification: RA644.A25 H48 1988 Dewey Class No.: 614.5/993 19

The Impending Catastrophe: a resource book on the emerging HIV/AIDS epidemic in South Africa / Henry J. Kaiser Family Foundation & LoveLife . Published/Created: Johannesburg: 2000. Description: 30p.

Third International Conference on Aids and Associated Cancers in Africa, reported as the second workshop for the East, Central, and Southern African Commonwealth Health Community held at the Arusha International Conference Centre, Arusha, Tanzania, September 14-16, 1988 / compiled by the Regional Health Secretary, Commonwealth Regional Health Community Secretariat. Published/Created: Arusha, Tanzania: The Secretariat, [1988 or 1989] Description: i, 9 p.; 29 cm.

Togni, Lorenzo S. AIDS in South Africa and on the African continent / Lorenzo Togni. Published/Created: Pretoria: Kagiso Publishers, c1997. Description: 109 p.: ill.; 21 cm. ISBN: 0798642149 Notes: Includes bibliographical

references (p. 89-90). Subjects: AIDS (Disease)--South Africa. AIDS (Disease)--Africa. LC Classification: RA644.A25 T633 1997 Dewey Class No.: 362.1/969792/00968 21 f-sa---

Torrey, Barbara Boyle. Blood donors and aids in Africa: the gift relationship revisited / by Barbara Boyle Torrey, Maurita Mulligan and Peter O. Way. Published/Created: Washington, D.C.: Center for International Research, U.S. Bureau of the Census, [1990] Related Authors: Mulligan, Maurita. Way, Peter O. Description: viii, 37 p.: ill.; 28 cm. Notes: Includes bibliographical references (p. 35-37). Subjects: AIDS (Disease)--Transmission--Africa. Blood--Transfusion--Safety measures. Series: CIR staff paper; no. 53 LC Classification: RC607.A26 T67 1990 Dewey Class No.: 616.97/92/0096 20

Unesco Regional Seminar on HIV/AIDS and Education within the School System for English-Speaking Countries in Eastern and Southern Africa (1995: Harare, Zimbabwe) Final report of the Unesco Regional Seminar on HIV/AIDS and Education within the School System for English-Speaking Countries in Eastern and

Southern Africa: 20 to 24 February 1995, Harare / convened by Unesco's Programme of Education for the Prevention of AIDS and the Education Programme of the Unesco Sub-Regional Office for Southern Africa in collaboration with the Swedish International Development Authority (SIDA) and World Health Organization/Global Programme on AIDS Regional Office for Africa. Published/Created: [Paris]: Unesco, Education Sector, c1995. Related Authors: Programme of Education for the Prevention of AIDS (Unesco) Unesco Sub-Regional Office for Southern Africa. Education Programme. Sweden. Styrelsen för internationell utveckling. Global Programme on AIDS (World Health Organization). Regional Office for Africa. Unesco. Education Sector. Description: 83 p.: ill. (some col.); 30 cm. Subjects: AIDS (Disease)--Africa, English-speaking--Prevention Congresses. AIDS (Disease)--Study and teaching--Africa, English-speaking--Congresses. LC Classification: RA643.86.A35 U64 1995

United States. Congress. House. Committee on Foreign Affairs. Subcommittee on Africa. Coping with AIDS in Africa:

three years into the W.H.O. program on AIDS: hearings before the Subcommittee on Africa of the Committee on Foreign Affairs, House of Representatives, One Hundred First Congress, first session, June 14 and July 19, 1989. Published/Created: Washington: U.S. G.P.O.: For sale by the Supt. of Docs., Congressional Sales Office, U.S. G.P.O., 1990. Description: iii, 121 p.: map; 23 cm. Notes: Distributed to some depository libraries in microfiche. Shipping list no.: 90-391-P. Item 1017-A, 1017-B (MF) Subjects: AIDS (Disease)--Africa, Sub-Saharan. Global Programme on AIDS (World Health Organization) LC Classification: KF27 .F625 1989c Dewey Class No.: 362.1/969792/0967 20 Govt. Doc. No.: Y 4.F 76/1:Ac 7 z Y 4.F 76/1:Aq 5/2

United States. Congress. House. Committee on Foreign Affairs. Subcommittee on Africa. The impact of HIV/AIDS on the social and economic development in Africa: hearing before the Subcommittee on Africa of the Committee on Foreign Affairs, House of Representatives, One Hundred Second Congress, first session, November 6, 1991. Published/Created: Washington:

U.S. G.P.O.: For sale by the U.S. G.P.O., Supt. of Docs., Congressional Sales Office, 1992. Description: iii, 106 p.: ill.; 23 cm. ISBN: 0160393760 Notes: Item 1017-A Item 1017-B (MF) Distributed to some depository libraries in microfiche. Shipping list no.: 93-0072-P. Includes bibliographical references. Subjects: HIV (Viruses)--Africa. AIDS (Disease)--Social aspects--Africa. AIDS (Disease)--Africa--Prevention. LC Classification: KF27 .F625 1991d Dewey Class No.: 303.48/5 20 Govt. Doc. No.: Y 4.F 76/1:H 88/61 n-us---

Vivekananda, Franklin. Shame has fallen on the earth - aids disease in Africa: socio-economic impact on the African nation / Franklin Vivekananda. Published/Created: Stockholm: Bethany Books, [1994] Description: 1 v. ISBN: 9186702386 LC Classification: ACQUISITION IN PROCESS

Vivre et penser le SIDA en Afrique = Experiencing and understanding AIDS in Africa / édité par Charles Becker ... [et al.] Parallel Experiencing and understanding AIDS in Africa Published/Created: Dakar: CODESRIA; Paris: Karthala: IRD, c1999. Related Authors:

Becker, Charles. Codesria. Institut de recherche pour le développement (France). Programme national de lutte contre le SIDA (Senegal). Description: 707 p.: ill., map; 24 cm. ISBN: 2865379450 Notes: Papers originally presented at an international symposium held in Sali Portudal, Senegal, November 4-8, 1996, organized jointly by CODESRIA, IRD, and PNLS. Includes bibliographical references. Papers in English or French. Subjects: AIDS (Disease)--Africa--Congresses. HIV infections--Africa--Congresses. Series: Hommes et sociétés. Variant Series: Collection "Hommes et sociétés" LC Classification: RA644.A25 V575 1999 Dewey Class No.: 362.1/969792/00968 21

Webb, Douglas, 1970- HIV and AIDS in Africa / Douglas Webb. Published/Created: London; Chicago: Pluto Press; Cape Town: David Philip; Pietermaritzburg; University of Natal Press, 1997. Description: xiii, 258 p.: ill.; 22 cm. ISBN: 0745311253 (hbk) Notes: Includes bibliographical references (p. [232]-250) and index.. Subjects: AIDS (Disease)--Africa. HIV Infections--epidemiology--

Africa. HIV Infections--
prevention & control--Africa.
LC Classification: RA644.A25
W39 1997 Dewey Class No.:
614.5/99392/0096 21

Whiteside, Alan. AIDS: the
challenge for South Africa /
Alan Whiteside and Clem
Sunter. Published/Created:

Cape Town: Human &
Rousseau, 2000. Related
Authors: Sunter, Clem, 1944-
Description: 179 p.: ill.; 22 cm.
Notes: Includes bibliographical
references (p. 169-179). Library
of Congress 101 Independence
Ave., SE Washington, DC
20540 EMAIL:
lconline@loc.gov

In: Aids in Africa: A Pandemic on the Move   ISBN 1-59454-596-0
Editor: Garson J. Claton, pp. 71-169   © 2006 Nova Science Publishers, Inc.

Chapter 4

BIBLIOGRAPHY–
JOURNALS AND MAGAZINES

ABNF J 2000 Jul-Aug;11(4):83-7
Community health, media, and policy in sub-Saharan Africa: a primary prevention approach to the AIDS crisis. Ndiwane AN. Bouve College of Health Sciences, School of Nursing, Northeastern University, USA. andiwane@lynx.neu.edu Availability, access and utilization of essential health services present challenges to community health services in Sub-Saharan Africa. HIV/AIDS infection has added yet another dimension to a continent already experiencing economic crises.

Acta Med Port 1999 Dec;12(12):367-70 Human immunodeficiency virus type 2 infection [Article in Portuguese] Mansinho K. Servico de Doencas Infecciosas, Hospital Egas Moniz, Lisboa. Controlled longitudinal studies suggest that the rate of progression to advanced HIV related disease and mortality are far lower for HIV-2 than for HIV-1. Understanding how, immunologically and virologically, HIV-2 behaves differently from HIV-1 may provide some insight into the mechanisms governing HIV-1 pathogenesis.

Acta Trop 1993 Sep;54(3-4):153-62 Current situation of African trypanosomiasis. Kuzoe FA. UNDP/WORLD BANK/WHO Special Programme for Research and Training in Tropical Diseases, World Health Organization, Geneva, Switzerland. African trypanosomiasis (sleeping sickness) is fatal, if untreated, and occurs in 36 African countries, south of the Sahara, where some 50 million people are at risk of acquiring infection. In view of the worsening economic situation of endemic countries, and the focus of attention and resources on the AIDS pandemic, prospects of any significant improvement in the sleeping sickness situation would largely depend on the successful mobilization of external resources.

Adv Parasitol 1998;40:399-418 Cyclospora cayetanensis. Ortega YR, Sterling CR, Gilman RH. Department of Veterinary Science and Microbiology, University of Arizona, Tucson, AZ 85721, USA. Cyclospora cayetanensis is a coccidian pathogen in humans. Cyclosporiasis is characterized by mild to severe nausea, anorexia, abdominal cramping, and watery diarrhea. Cyclospora infections can be treated successfully with trimethoprim-sulfamethoxazole.

Adv Pediatr Infect Dis 1993;8:145-57 The acquired immunodeficiency syndrome (AIDS) in African children. Goldfarb J. Division of Infectious Disease, Rainbow Babies and Childrens Hospital,

Cleveland, Ohio.

Adv Tech Stand Neurosurg 1994;21:155-82 AIDS and the neurosurgeon--an update. Ciricillo SF, Rosenblum ML. Department of Neurological Surgery, School of Medicine, University of California, San Francisco. Over the past decade, acquired immunodeficiency syndrome (AIDS) has become the leading public health crisis in the United States, Western Europe, and Africa. Despite improvements in the diagnosis and treatment of AIDS-related disorders, the number of people infected with the human immunodeficiency virus (HIV-1) continues to grow, requiring a greater proportion of limited financial, medical, and human resources.

Adv Virus Res 1999;53:71-88 Human immunodeficiency viruses in the developing world. Essex M. Harvard AIDS Institute, Harvard School of Public Health, Boston, Massachusetts 02115-6017, USA. AIDS has become a major burden in developing countries. At present, more than 90% of new HIV infections are emerging in Asia and Africa. Particularly ominous is the epidemic due to HIV-1 C in southern Africa, where about

25% of adults in several countries are infected. Although most of its spread apparently occurred during the 1990s, HIV-1 C currently accounts for one-half of the infections in the world.

Afr Dent J. 1993;7:11-9 HIV infection in children: a challenge to dental practice. Sote EO. Department of Child Dental Health, College of Medicine, University of Lagos. Human immunodeficiency virus infection in children is on the increase globally. Because of diagnostic difficulties of HIV infection in children, among other reasons, all children are suspects. As a result of new developments in the treatment of this condition, more people with HIV infection/AIDS will survive and require dental treatment on a long-term basis.

AIDS 1996 Dec;10 Suppl 3:S61-7 HIV/AIDS in resource-poor settings: comprehensive care across a continuum. Osborne CM. Department of Paediatrics and Child Health, University Teaching Hospital, Lusaka, Zambia. BACKGROUND: The scale of the HIV pandemic in many resource-poor settings (RPS) has overwhelmed the already impoverished health and social support systems.

OBJECTIVE: To propose a feasible and applicable model of care which can be used at district level in RPS faced with the prospect of caring for increasing numbers of persons living with HIV and AIDS (PWA) requiring care, and to outline some of the immediate challenges and directions for research.

AIDS 1996 Jun;10(7):689-99 Lessons from the second AIDS virus, HIV-2. Marlink R.

AIDS 1996;10 Suppl A:S205-11 The socioeconomic impact of AIDS in sub-Saharan Africa. Chevallier E, Floury D. Joint United Nations Programme on HIV/AIDS, Geneva, Switzerland.

AIDS 1997 Dec;11(15):17-36 HIV-1 subtypes: implications for epidemiology, pathogenicity, vaccines and diagnostics. Workshop Report from the European Commission (DG XII, INCO-DC) and the Joint United Nations Programme on HIV/AIDS. Forty-three AIDS scientists from Europe, Africa, the United States, Canada, India and China met in Dar es Salaam, Tanzania to discuss the implications of the global variation of HIV (list of participants included in

Appendix). Key elements of the discussion are summarized here in the context of a review of the current literature.

AIDS 1997;11 Suppl A:S217-25 Comment in: AIDS. 1997 ;11 Suppl A:S181-2 Involving traditional healers in AIDS education and counselling in sub-Saharan Africa: a review. King R, Homsy J. Medecins Sans Frontieres-Switzerland in Kampala, Uganda.

AIDS 1997;11 Suppl B:S115-23 Tuberculosis and HIV: current status in Africa. Raviglione MC, Harries AD, Msiska R, Wilkinson D, Nunn P. Global Tuberculosis Programme, World Health Organization, Geneva, Switzerland.

AIDS 1997;11 Suppl B:S125-34 Care of children with HIV infection and AIDS in Africa. Marum LH, Tindyebwa D, Gibb D. John Hopkins University, Baltimore, Maryland, USA.

AIDS 1997;11 Suppl B:S143-9 Government responses to HIV/AIDS in Africa: what have we learnt? Abdool Karim Q, Tarantola D, As Sy E, Moodie R. Southern African HIV/AIDS International Training and Research Programme, c/o Medical Research Council,

Pretoria, South Africa. While we should not lose sight of the development of vaccines and cures, more immediate priorities include the implementation of effective STD control. The syndromic management approach developed in Zimbabwe to overcome laboratory constraints is a cost-effective way of managing STD. Of urgency is the integration of STD services into primary health-care services, appropriate training of staff, adequate provision and control over drugs and condoms, and incorporation of traditional healers and community-based education on STD. A second area of priority is the strengthening of the interaction between prevention, care and support activities, which act in synergy.

AIDS 1997;11 Suppl B:S159-67 A human rights perspective on HIV/AIDS in sub-Saharan Africa. Gruskin S, Wakhweya AM. Human Rights Program, Francois-Xavier Bagnoud Center for Health and Human Rights, Harvard School of Public Health, Boston, MA 02115, USA.

AIDS 1997;11 Suppl B:S43-54 Natural history and spectrum of disease in adults with HIV/AIDS in Africa. Grant AD,

Djomand G, De Cock KM. Project RETRO-CI, Abidjan, Cote d'Ivoire. Progression from seroconversion to the development of AIDS in Africa may be shorter than in industrialized countries, but there are insufficient data to be certain. Although the data are not always directly comparable, survival after an AIDS diagnosis appears to be substantially shorter in African countries and this may be partly because of later diagnosis of AIDS in Africa, but may also be because of environmental factors such as increased exposure to pathogens of high virulence and lack of access to care. Tuberculosis and bacterial infections are the most important causes of morbidity and mortality among hospitalized patients. The most important research questions concern the development and evaluation of cost-effective regimes for prophylaxis and treatment of opportunistic disease in order to prolong healthy life in HIV-infected individuals.

AIDS 1997;11 Suppl B:S5-21 HIV/AIDS epidemics in sub-Saharan Africa: dynamism, diversity and discrete declines? Tarantola D, Schwartlander B. International AIDS Program of the Francois-Xavier Bagnoud Center for Health and Human Rights, Harvard School of Public Health, Boston, MA 02115, USA.

AIDS 1997;11 Suppl B:S55-61 The demographic and economic impact of AIDS in Africa. Whiteside A, Stover J. Economic Research Unit, University of Natal, Durban.

AIDS 1997;11 Suppl B:S99-106 The challenge of providing effective care for HIV/AIDS in Africa. Gilks CF, Katabira E, De Cock KM. Liverpool School of Tropical Medicine, UK.

AIDS 1998;12 Suppl 1:S15-27 Impact of the HIV epidemic on mortality in sub-Saharan Africa: evidence from national surveys and censuses. Timaeus IM. Centre for Population Studies, London School of Hygiene and Tropical Medicine, UK. OBJECTIVE: To measure recent trends in all-cause child and adult mortality in national populations in sub-Saharan Africa. CONCLUSIONS: Data can be collected in national household surveys and censuses to monitor the mortality impact of HIV in Africa. Such data have begun to document the differential impact of the epidemic. In those countries with data in which HIV became prevalent by the late 1980s, massive rises in adult mortality occurred by the mid-1990s.

AIDS 1998;12 Suppl 1:S29-39 Projecting the impact of AIDS on mortality. Stover J, Way P. Futures Group International, Glastonbury, Connecticut 06033, USA. OBJECTIVE: To illustrate the magnitude of the impact of AIDS on projections of mortality, to explain the reasons for the differences in projections by major international organizations and to provide a simple approach to estimating the impact of AIDS on life expectancy.

AIDS 1998;12 Suppl 1:S3-14 Mortality impact of the AIDS epidemic: evidence from community studies in less developed countries. Boerma JT, Nunn AJ, Whitworth JA. Carolina Population Center, University of North Carolina at Chapel Hill 27516, USA. BACKGROUND: The AIDS epidemic is now more than a decade old and direct evidence of mortality impact has become measurable, as indicated by an increasing number of publications presenting empirical data from less developed countries.

AIDS 1999 Feb 4;13(2):IAS1-3

Place of antiretroviral drugs in the treatment of HIV-infected people in Africa. International AIDS Society.

AIDS 2000 Jun 16;14(9):1091-9 Prevention of infectious complications of paediatric HIV infection in Africa. Dray-Spira R, Lepage P, Dabis F.

AIDS 2000 Sep 29;14(14):2071-81 Concurrent infections and HIV pathogenesis. Bentwich Z, Maartens G, Torten D, Lal AA, Lal RB. Ruth Ben-Ari Institute of Clinical Immunology & AIDS Center, Kaplan Medical Center, Hebrew University Hadassah Medical School, Rehovot, Israel.

AIDS 2000;14 Suppl 3:S239-52 Economic costs of HIV/AIDS prevention activities in sub-Saharan Africa. Kumaranayake L, Watts C. Health Policy Unit, London School of Hygiene and Tropical Medicine, UK.

AIDS 2000;14 Suppl 3:S275-84 A review of current literature on the impact of HIV/AIDS on children in sub-Saharan Africa. Foster G, Williamson J. Family AIDS Caring Trust, Mutare, Zimbabwe.

AIDS 2001 Jan 26;15(2):143-52 Tuberculosis case fatality rates in high HIV prevalence populations in sub-Saharan Africa. Mukadi YD, Maher D, Harries A. BACKGROUND: Tuberculosis is a leading cause worldwide of morbidity and mortality among HIV-infected people. The HIV era has seen a dramatic increase of the tuberculosis case fatality rate (CFR) in high HIV prevalence populations. Providing care for HIV-infected people must include measures to tackle this high tuberculosis CFR. AIMS: To analyse the extent of the increased tuberculosis CFR in high HIV prevalence populations in sub-Saharan Africa, the reasons for this increase and the causes of death, in order to identify possible ways of tackling this problem.

AIDS Care 1993;5(1):5-22 The impact of HIV/AIDS on the family and other significant relationships: the African clan revisited. Ankrah EM. Faculty of Social Sciences, Makerere University, Kampala, Uganda. Although changing in size, structure and function, the African family has persistently maintained its place as the central human social unit. Beyond the traditional African family--whether in the nuclear or the extended form--is a network of people, most of whom are connected by kin or blood relationships, termed the clanship system. Patterns of family treatment and care are deeply embedded in this wider kinship system.

AIDS Care 1995;7(3):365-73 Women and AIDS in Zambia: a review of the psychosocial factors implicated in the transmission of HIV. Campbell T, Kelly M. Hillingdon Hospital, Uxbridge, Middlesex, UK. Women are at high risk for HIV infection in Zambia. There are several interrelated factors to account for this including the economic, cultural and educational status of women. This paper explores these factors and suggests that these factors need to be thoroughly understood before preventive strategies are designed and implemented.

AIDS Patient Care STDS 1998 Jun;12(6):435-49 The basic reproductive rate of infection and the course of HIV epidemics. Garnett GP. Wellcome Trust Centre for the Epidemiology of Infectious Disease University of Oxford, England. The basic reproductive rate is a measure of the potential for growth of an infectious disease epidemic and depends on the pattern of infectious contacts within the host population, the likelihood of infection being transmitted during a contact, and the duration of infectiousness. These three variables are reviewed along with the surveillance data that records the progress of the epidemic, with an emphasis on the HIV-1 epidemic in heterosexual populations in developing countries.

AIDS Patient Care STDS 1999 Aug;13(8):459-65 Kala-azar as an AIDS-related opportunistic infection. Murray HW. Department of Medicine, Cornell University Medical College, New York, New York, USA. Visceral leishmaniasis (kala-azar) is a worldwide disseminated protozoal infection primarily transmitted by sand flies. Because host defense against this intracellular infection is T-cell-dependent, kala-azar has predictably joined the list of AIDS-related opportunistic infections in endemic areas. The vast majority of patients with AIDS-associated kala-azar are currently found in southern Europe (the Mediterranean basin, especially Spain in injection drug users); future cases will inevitably arise in other endemic regions including India, East Africa and Sudan, and Brazil. Optimal primary and secondary prophylaxis for AIDS-related kala-azar remain to be determined; life-long maintenance therapy is becoming an accepted approach.

AIDS Patient Care STDS 1999 Dec;13(12):717-30 Heterosexual anal intercourse: prevalence, cultural factors, and HIV infection and other health risks, Part I. Halperin DT. International Center for HIV/AIDS Research and Clinical Training in Nursing, University of California, San Francisco, USA. dhalp@itsa.ucsf.edu Studies of heterosexual HIV transmission have consistently found anal intercourse to be a highly predictive risk factor for seroconversion. Yet most AIDS prevention messages targeted at heterosexuals, presumably influenced by cultural taboos against acknowledging this sexual practice, continue to emphasize vaginal and, increasingly, oral sex transmission. The health risks of anal sex appear to be severely underestimated by a substantial proportion of sexually active women and men in North and Latin America as well as parts of South Asia, Africa, and other regions. This typically stigmatized and hidden sexual practice must be given greater emphasis in AIDS/STD prevention, women's care, and other health promotion programs.

AIDS Res Hum Retroviruses 1998 Oct;14 Suppl 3:S321-3 Rationale for the testing and use of a partially effective HIV vaccine. Vermund SH. School of Public Health, University of Alabama at Birmingham, 35294-2170, USA. sten@uab.edu

Am J Epidemiol 1998 Feb 1;147(3):217-21 Kaposi's sarcoma (KS), KS-associated herpesvirus, and the criteria for causality in the age of molecular biology. Moore PS, Chang Y. Division of Epidemiology, School of Public Health, Columbia University, New York, NY 10032, USA.

Am J Public Health 1997 Dec;87(12):1917-9 Comment on: Am J Public Health. 1997 Dec;87(12):1931-6. Good news for everyone? Stanton B.

Am J Trop Med Hyg 1996 Jul;55(1):1-11 Preventing opportunistic infections in human immunodeficiency virus-infected persons: implications for the developing world.

Kaplan JE, Hu DJ, Holmes KK, Jaffe HW, Masur H, De Cock KM. Division of AIDS, STD, and TB Laboratory Research, National Center for Infectious Diseases, Centers for Disease Control and Prevention, Atlanta, Georgia, USA. More than 18 million persons in the world are estimated to have been infected with human immunodeficiency virus (HIV), the cause of the acquired immunodeficiency syndrome (AIDS). As immunodeficiency progresses, these persons become susceptible to a wide variety of opportunistic infections (OIs) The spectrum of OIs varies among regions of the world. An increasing problem in the developing world, HIV/AIDS should receive attention comparable to other tropical diseases.

Am J Trop Med Hyg 1998 Mar;58(3):273-6 The historical question of acquired immunodeficiency syndrome in the 1960s in the Congo River basin area in relation to cryptococcal meningitis. Molez JF. Laboratoire de Paludologie, Institut Francais de Recherche Scientifique pour le Developpement en Cooperation (ORSTOM), Dakar, Senegal. In Europe before the advent of the acquired immunodeficiency syndrome (AIDS), fatal cases of infection with Cryptococcus neoformans resembling acute meningitis were rarely described and never in young adults. However, rapidly fatal cryptococcal meningitis in young Africans has been known to exist in central Africa for at least 30 years, mainly in the lower area of the Congo River basin.

Am J Trop Med Hyg 2001 Dec;65(6):810-21 Preventing opportunistic infections among human immunodeficiency virus-infected adults in African countries. Grant AD, Kaplan JE, De Cock KM. Clinical Research Unit, London School of Hygiene and Tropical Medicine, London, United Kingdom. The burden of human immunodeficiency virus (HIV)-related disease in sub-Saharan Africa continues to increase; providing adequate care for the huge number of people affected is a daunting task, especially given the limited resources available. Recent studies have shown that low-cost regimens can prevent some of the most important causes of HIV-related disease in African countries. The availability of effective and affordable regimens to prevent HIV-related disease may also encourage people to seek HIV testing, combat denial, and help overcome the sense of powerlessness in countries where the HIV epidemic has hit hardest.

Ann Cardiol Angeiol (Paris) 1997 Feb;46(2):81-7 The effect of HIV infection on high incidence of heart diseases in Kinshass (Zaire). Echocardiographic study [Article in French] Longo-Mbenza B, Tonduangu K, Kintonki Vita E, Seghers KV. Service de Cardiologie, Universite de Kinshasa, Zare. Invasion of the heart by HIV has become a clinical problem over the last decade. The objective of the present study was to systematically detect the excess HIV-related cardiac lesions in Kinshasa by performing echocardiography.

Ann Intern Med 1993 Feb 1;118(3):211-8 Infection with the human immunodeficiency virus type 2. Markovitz DM. University of Michigan Medical Center, Ann Arbor. PURPOSE: To review the clinical, epidemiologic, and biological features of infection with the human immunodeficiency virus type 2 (HIV-2).

Ann Med Interne (Paris) 1994;145(6):424-8 African histoplasmosis: clinical and therapeutic aspects, relation to AIDS. Apropos of 4 cases, including a case with HIV-1-HTLV-1 co-infection [Article in French] Geffray L, Veyssier P, Cevallos R, Beaud B, Mayolle J, Nogier C, Ray E, Thouvenot D. Service de Medecine Interne et Maladies Infectieuses, Centre Hospitalier de Compiegne, Compiegne. The authors report 4 cases of African histoplasmosis in Zairans.

Ann N Y Acad Sci 1992 Jun 16;653:257-73 Macroepidemiology of the HIVs-AIDS (HAIDS) pandemic. Insufficiently considered zoological and geopolitical aspects. Torres-Anjel MJ. Department of Microbiology (Clinical Epidemiology), College of Veterinary Medicine, University of Missouri, Columbia. The human immunodeficiency viruses (HIVs)-acquired immunodeficiency syndrome (AIDS) or HAIDS pandemic originated from lentiviruses of nonhuman primates (thus qualifying as a zoonosis) that moved into humans in Africa.

Ann N Y Acad Sci 2000 Nov;918:128-35 Psychosocial and community perspectives on alternatives to breastfeeding. Bassett MT. Department of

Community Medicine, University of Zimbabwe Medical School, Avondale, Harare, Zimbabwe. mary@zappuz.co.zw In developing countries, what advice to give HIV-positive mothers on infant feeding options remains a vexing public health issue. This paper reviews data on infant feeding practices in sub-Saharan Africa, the cultural context of breastfeeding, and the still meager literature of decision-making by HIV-positive mothers, following impartial counseling. By offering actual feeding choices to HIV-positive women, observing what choices they make, and monitoring the outcomes of these choices, we will be better placed to give advice.

Ann N Y Acad Sci 2000 Nov;918:156-62 Mastitis and transmission of human immunodeficiency virus through breast milk. Semba RD. Ocular Immunology Service, Johns Hopkins University School of Medicine, Baltimore, Maryland, USA. Mastitis, an inflammation in the breast, has recently been linked with higher human immunodeficiency virus (HIV) load in breast milk and higher risk of mother-to-child transmission of HIV.

Ann N Y Acad Sci 2000 Nov;918:330-45 Rapid characterization of HIV clade C-specific cytotoxic T lymphocyte responses in infected African children and adults. Goulder PJ. Partners AIDS Research Center, Massachusetts General Hospital, Charlestown, Massachusetts 02129, USA. goulder@helix.mgh.harvard.edu Cytotoxic T lymphocytes (CTL) play a central role in successful control of HIV. Induction of effective CTL responses may therefore be an essential requirement of HIV vaccines. Knowledge of CTL epitopes targeted either in natural infection or following vaccination will be critical to understanding the anti-HIV immune response. This review summarizes the evidence that cellular immunity is important in successful containment of HIV and describes the novel methods of epitope detection, illustrating their ready application to the study of C-clade infected persons in sub-Saharan Africa.

Ann N Y Acad Sci 2000 Nov;918:57-63 Access to voluntary counseling and testing for HIV in developing countries. Coovadia HM. Department of Paediatrics and Child Health,
Faculty of Medicine, University of Natal, Private Bag X7, Congella, South Africa 4013. The counseling that precedes and follows testing of subjects for HIV has become, quite unexpectedly, a focal point for assessment of the ethical propriety, availability, and appropriateness of health services during the AIDS epidemic. Obstacles to be overcome for provision of VCCT services are identified. Evidence for a positive impact of VCCT services includes facilitated decision-making, acceptance and coping with HIV, improved family and community acceptance, increased condom use, and reduced gonorrhea rates and HIV transmission.

Ann N Y Acad Sci 2001 Nov;946:1-12 The changing picture of the HIV/AIDS epidemic. Ippolito G, Galati V, Serraino D, Girardi E. Dipartimento di Epidemiologia, Istituto Nazionale per le Malattie Infettive Lazzaro Spallanzani-IRCCS, Rome, Italy. ippolito@inmi.it Twenty years after it was first recognized, the HIV/AIDS epidemic continues to expand, but its impact varies greatly in different parts of the World. The worst of the epidemic is now centered in developing countries, especially sub-Saharan Africa, and areas such as Eastern Europe, which was only marginally involved a few years ago but has recently experienced the largest growth in the epidemic. Interventions addressed to encourage the adoption of safer sex practices are badly needed, since a "rebound" in risky sexual behaviors was recently reported among high risk groups, which is, at least in part, attributable to the optimism about new treatments.

Arch Dis Child 1995 Apr;72(4):369-74 The challenge of diagnosing childhood tuberculosis in a developing country. Osborne CM. University Teaching Hospital, Department of Paediatrics and Child Health, Lusaka, Zambia.

Arch Dis Child 1998 Sep;79(3):274-8 Ethambutol in tuberculosis: time to reconsider? Graham SM, Daley HM, Banerjee A, Salaniponi FM, Harries AD. College of Medicine, University of Malawi, Chichiri, Malawi. sgraham@unima.wn.apc.org

Arch Inst Pasteur Alger 1998;62:201-14 Pneumocystis carinii pneumopathy in patients with AIDS. The first 3 cases reported in Algeria and review of the literature [Article in French] Mansouri R, Abed-Benamara M. Laboratoire de Parasitologie-Mycologie CHU Mustapha. Pneumocystis carinii pneumonia (PCP) is a severe and dangerous infection which afflicts patients with immune deficiency, particularly those with AIDS. This pathology isn't well known in Algeria. The aim of the present study is a contribution to make this disease more known in the algerian AIDS patients.

Arch Ophthalmol 1997 Oct;115(10):1291-5 HIV and AIDS and the eye in developing countries: a review. Lewallen S, Courtright P. Department of Ophthalmology, University of British Columbia, St Paul's Hospital, Vancouver, Canada. An estimated 30 million people worldwide have been infected with the human immunodeficiency virus, the causative agent of the acquired immunodeficiency syndrome. Of these, 90% live in developing countries from where there is relatively little published information about the ocular manifestations of human immunodeficiency virus and acquired immunodeficiency syndrome. We review the information available from

Africa, Latin America, and Asia.

Arch Virol Suppl 1996;11:195-202 HIV-1 subtype O: epidemiology, pathogenesis, diagnosis, and perspectives of the evolution of HIV. Gurtler LG, Zekeng L, Tsague JM, van Brunn A, Afane Ze E, Eberle J, Kaptue L. Max von Pettenkofer Institute for Hygiene and Medical Microbiology, University of Munich, Federal Republic of Germany. HIV-1 subtype O is a new HIV variant originating in the West-Central African region, with highest prevalences in countries such as Cameroon, Equatorial Guinea and Gabon. Detection of antibodies to HIV-1 subtype O can pose problems in unmodified ELISA tests, and confirmation of anti-HIV-1 subtype O in immunoblot may give false negative results in some specimens. Nucleic acid-based assays designed for HIV-1 detection do not amplify or detect sequences from HIV-1 subtype O. In their env sequences, HIV-1 subtype O strains show a higher heterogeneity than the classical HIV-1 subtypes, leading to the conclusion that HIV-1 subtype O has been introduced into the human population only recently. Further, unidentified subtypes are also likely to exist.

Aust J Rural Health 2001 Aug;9(4):158-65 Fostering hope in people living with AIDS in Africa: the role of primary health-care workers. Akinsola HA. Department of Nursing Education, University of Botswana, Gaborone, Botswana. akinsola@mopipi.ub.bw Today the medical literature is dominated by discussions on issues related to HIV/AIDS. This is not surprising considering the fact that in the history of humankind, the HIV/AIDS scenario has posed one of the greatest challenges. The reality of the physical, socioeconomic and psychological problems associated with the AIDS epidemic has become obvious to the general populace in Africa.

Baillieres Best Pract Res Clin Rheumatol 2000 Sep;14(3):579-93 Rheumatic manifestations of HIV-AIDS. Cuellar ML, Espinoza LR. Section of Rheumatology, Department of Medicine, Tulane University Medical Center, 1415 Tulane Avenue, New Orleans, LA, 70112, USA. Infection by human immunodeficiency virus is characterized by a myriad of clinical manifestations affecting almost every organ system in the body. If untreated, it follows an inexorable course, leading to a profound state of immunosuppression and eventually death from opportunistic infection and/or development of lymphoproliferative malignancy and Kaposi's sarcoma. Rheumatic manifestations may develop at any time of the clinical spectrum, but usually are more often seen in late stages.

Baillieres Clin Haematol 1992 Apr;5(2):273-314 Human retroviruses. Weber T, Hunsmann G, Stevens W, Fleming AF. It was only in 1980 that the first human retrovirus, HTLV-1, was isolated. Since then, HTLV-2, HIV-1 and HIV-2 have been identified. All four viruses are transmitted with varying efficiency sexually, vertically from mother to infant, and through blood by transfusion or contamination.

Biologist (London) 2001 Apr;48(2):64-6 HIV: vaccines out of Africa. Rowland-Jones S. Human Immunology Unit, Institute of Molecular Medicine, John Radcliffe Hospital, Headington, Oxford, OX3 9DS, UK. When HIV was first identified as the cause of AIDS in 1983, it was widely expected that a vaccine would be relatively straightforward to make. Why, eighteen years later, are we still waiting?

Biometrics 1994 Dec;50(4):899-916 The world of biometry. Billard L. Department of Statistics, University of Georgia, Athens 30602-1952, USA. The International Biometric Society is an international society for the advancement of biological science through the development of quantitative theories and the application, development and dissemination of effective mathematical and statistical techniques. We consider some of the nonscientific and scientific issues being addressed by researchers in and across Regions and Groups of our Biometric world. These run the gamut of theoretical to applied mathematics and statistics with the applications spanning many fields and, not surprisingly, forming a rich source of new theoretical developments.

BMJ 2002 Jan 26;324(7331):226-9 First trial of the HIV-1 vaccine in Africa: Ugandan experience. Mugerwa RD, Kaleebu P, Mugyenyi P, Katongole-Mbidde E, Hom DL, Byaruhanga R, Salata RA, Ellner JJ; HIV-1 Vaccine Trial Group.

Department of Medicine,
Makerere University Medical
School, Kampala, Uganda.
profrdm@imul.com

BMJ 2002 Jan 26;324(7331):232-4
The impact of HIV and AIDS
on Africa's economic
development. Dixon S,
McDonald S, Roberts J. School
of Health and Related Research,
University of Sheffield,
Sheffield S1 4DA, UK.
S.Dixon@shef.ac.uk

Br J Hosp Med 1992 Dec 2-1993
Jan 5;48(11):734-7, 740-1
Clinical manifestations of
African AIDS. Kelly MP.
Monze District Hospital,
Zambia. AIDS (acquired
immunodeficiency syndrome) is
now the greatest cause of death
in many African countries. Any
traveller from sub-Saharan
Africa may present with an
AIDS-related condition. This
article provides a brief
introduction to the problems
posed by AIDS and AIDS-
related conditions and their
recognition.

Br J Ophthalmol 2001
Aug;85(8):897-903 Blindness
in Africa: present situation and
future needs. Lewallen S,
Courtright P. British Columbia
Centre for Epidemiologic and
International Ophthalmology.

AIM: To review the prevalence
and causes of blindness in sub-
Saharan Africa, the existing
services and limitations, and the
Vision 2020 goals for the future.
CONCLUSIONS: Blindness
prevalence rates vary widely but
the evidence suggests that
approximately 1% of Africans
are blind. The major cause is
cataract; trachoma and
glaucoma are also important
causes of blindness. The bulk of
blindness in the region is
preventable or curable. Efforts
should focus on eye problems
which are universally present
and for which there are cost
effective remedies, such as
cataract and refractive problems
and on those problems which
occur focally and can be
prevented by primary healthcare
measures, such as trachoma,
onchocerciasis, and vitamin A
deficiency. Major development
of staffing levels, infrastructure,
and community programmes
will be necessary to achieve
Vision 2020 goals.

Br J Surg 1997 Jan;84(1):8-14
Surgery for tuberculosis before
and after human
immunodeficiency virus
infection: a tropical perspective.
Watters DA. AIM: To review
from a tropical perspective the
presentation and management of
tuberculosis and how it is

affected by coexistent human immunodeficiency virus (HIV) infection. CONCLUSION: All surgeons need to be aware of the manifestations of tuberculosis at different sites and the effects of HIV infection. HIV-positive patients are more likely to present with systemic illness and multiple sites of involvement, and to respond poorly to major surgery. Surgical management is generally limited to making a diagnosis or treating life-threatening complications.

Br Med Bull 1996 Oct;52(4):682-703 Geographic and ethnic variations in the incidence of childhood cancer. Stiller CA, Parkin DM. Childhood Cancer Research Group, University of Oxford, UK. The total incidence of childhood cancer varies rather little between different regions of the world, with cumulative risk to age 15 nearly always in the range 1.0-2.5 per thousand. Acute lymphoblastic leukaemia, especially in early childhood, is most common in populations of high socio-economic status and is the most frequent childhood cancer in all industrialised countries. The risk of Burkitt's lymphoma is highest in tropical Africa and Papua New Guinea; it is strongly associated with Epstein-Barr

virus infection and intense immune stimulation by malaria. Other lymphomas are also relatively common in developing countries.

Br Med Bull 1998;54(2):383-93 Acute bacterial infections and HIV disease. Gilks CF. Liverpool School of Tropical Medicine, UK. Some acute bacterial infections, notably those caused by the pneumococcus and the non-typhi salmonellae, have not traditionally been considered as leading diseases in tropical medicine, despite their ubiquitous distribution and impact on health. The HIV/AIDS epidemic is forcing a re-evaluation of this position because of their importance in immunosuppressed adults, particularly where exposure is high and treatment relatively inadequate.

Br Med Bull 2001;58:7-18 The global epidemiology of HIV/AIDS. Morison L. MRC Tropical Epidemiology Group, Infectious Disease Epidemiology Unit, Department of Infectious and Tropical Diseases, London School of Hygiene and Tropical Medicine, London, UK. In this paper, the ways in which HIV is transmitted and factors facilitating transmission are described, although we still do not fully understand why the HIV epidemic has spread so heterogeneously across the globe. Estimates of HIV prevalence vary in quality but give some idea of trends in different countries and regions. Of all regions in the world, sub-Saharan Africa is the hardest hit by HIV, containing around 70% of people living with HIV/AIDS. There are, however, recent signs of hope in Africa due to a slight reduction in the number of new HIV cases in the year 2000.

Br Med Bull 2001;58:73-88 Demography and economics of HIV/AIDS. Whiteside A. Health Economics and HIV/AIDS Research Division, University of Natal, Durban, South Africa. The rapid spread of HIV in the 1980s and 1990s in the non-industrialised world is now leading to an AIDS epidemic. This in turn is having a demographic and economic impact on these societies. This article assesses the most recent evidence for these impacts. It concludes that, while there is already a real and measurable impact, there is far worse to come.

Br Med Bull 2001;58:89-108

Pediatric HIV infection: correlates of protective immunity and global perspectives in prevention and management. Goulder PJ, Jeena P, Tudor-Williams G, Burchett S. Partners AIDS Research Center, Massachusetts General Hospital, Harvard Medical School, Charlestown, Massachusetts 02129, USA. The impact of the HIV epidemic on child health globally is beginning to be appreciated. With the burden of new infections falling on young women, there is a skyrocketing number of AIDS orphans, and a rapidly increasing number of children infected via mother-to-child-transmission (MTCT). An estimated 600,000 new pediatric infections occur each year, of which some 1500/day (> 90%) occur in sub-Saharan Africa.

Bull Acad Natl Med 1993 Oct;177(7):1131-48; discussion 1149-52 Comparative epidemiology of HTLV and HIV retroviruses [Article in French] Tuppin P, de The G. Unite d'Epidemiologie des Virus Oncogenes, Institut Pasteur, Paris. There are interesting contrasts between the epidemiological characteristics of the two subfamilies of human retroviruses. The oncoretrovirus HTLV-I and II are endemic in

Intertropical Africa, North and South Americas and in the South of Japan. The lentiretroviruses HIV 1 and 2 are epidemic in the five continents and are progressing rapidly.

Bull Soc Pathol Exot 1996;89(4):282-6 Diffuse cutaneous leishmaniasis and acquired immunodeficiency syndrome in a Senegalese patient [Article in French] Ndiaye PB, Develoux M, Dieng MT, Huerre M. Clinique dermatologique, CHU Le Dantee, Dakar, Senegal. Tegumentary leishmaniasis cases associated with HIV infections were rarely reported. We present a case of diffuse cutaneous leishmaniasis in a senegalese patient with HIV 1 infection. The diagnosis was supported by a cutaneous biopsy but no Leishmania strain could be isolated by cultures from cutaneous specimens.

Bull Soc Pathol Exot 1999 Sep-Oct;92(4):261-3 Variability of human immunodeficiency virus type 1 [Article in French] Brun-Vezinet F, Damond F, Simon F. Laboratoire de virologie, Hopital Bichat-Claude Bernard, Paris, France. The variability of human immunodeficiency virus type 1 (HIV-1) is very high. To date, three distinct lineages of HIVs, type 1 group M, type 1 group O and type 2 are described, suggesting at least three different zoonotic infections. HIV-1 group M is responsible for the global epidemic of AIDS. At least ten subtypes of HIV-1 group M, labelled A through J, have been discovered. Viral sequences from both the gag and the env gene, particularly a part of gp 120 referred to as the V3 region have been used to identify subtypes of HIV-1 group M.

Bull World Health Organ 1997;75(5):477-89 Practical and affordable measures for the protection of health care workers from tuberculosis in low-income countries. Harries AD, Maher D, Nunn P. College of Medicine, University of Malawi, Chichiri. With the global upsurge in tuberculosis (TB), fueled by the human immunodeficiency virus (HIV) pandemic, and the increase in multidrug-resistant TB, the condition has become a serious occupational hazard for health care workers worldwide. Much of the current understanding about nosocomial TB transmission stems from the USA; however, little is known about the risk of such transmission in low-income countries. The focus of this review is on sub-Saharan Africa, since this is the region with the highest TB incidence, the highest HIV incidence, the worst epidemic of HIV-related TB, and where the risk to health care workers is probably greatest.

Bull World Health Organ 1998;76(6):651-62 An approach to the problems of diagnosing and treating adult smear-negative pulmonary tuberculosis in high-HIV-prevalence settings in sub-Saharan Africa. Harries AD, Maher D, Nunn P. College of Medicine, Chichiri, Blantyre, Malawi. The overlap between the populations in sub-Saharan Africa infected with human immunodeficiency virus (HIV) and Mycobacterium tuberculosis has led to an upsurge in tuberculosis cases over the last 10 years. The relative increase in the proportion of notified sputum-smear-negative pulmonary tuberculosis (PTB) cases is greater than that of sputum-smear-positive PTB cases. This is a consequence of the following: the association between decreased host immunity and reduced sputum smear positivity; the difficulty in excluding other HIV-related diseases when making the

diagnosis of smear-negative PTB; and an increase in false-negative sputum smears because of overstretched resources. This article examines problems in the diagnosis and treatment of smear-negative PTB in high-HIV-prevalence areas in sub-Saharan Africa.

Bull World Health Organ 2001;79(6):569-77 Targeted interventions required against genital ulcers in African countries worst affected by HIV infection. O'Farrell N. ofarrell@postmaster.co.uk It remains unclear why there is such marked variation in the severity of the human immunodeficiency virus (HIV) epidemic between African countries. The prevalence of HIV infection has reached high levels in many parts of southern Africa but in most countries of West Africa the levels are much lower. Although there is good evidence that sexually transmitted infections (STIs) and genital ulcers in particular facilitate heterosexual transmission of HIV, there is little comparative STI data from the African countries worst affected by HIV infection. A MEDLINE search covering the period 1966 to August 2000 using the keywords "sexually transmitted diseases", "genital ulcers" and "Africa" was performed to identify factors that might be relevant to the spread of HIV infection in countries with the highest prevalences of the virus.

C R Acad Sci III 1999 Nov;322(11):959-66 New prospects for the development of a vaccine against human immunodeficiency virus type 1. An overview. Girard M, Habel A, Chanel C. Departement de virologie, Institut Pasteur, Paris, France. mgirard@pasteur.fr During the past few years, definite progress has been made in the field of human immunodeficiency virus type 1 (HIV-1) vaccines. Initial attempts using envelope gp120 or gp140 from T-cell line-adapted (TCLA) HIV-1 strains to vaccinate chimpanzees showed that neutralizing antibody-based immune responses were protective against challenge with homologous TCLA virus strains or strains with low replicative capacity, but these neutralizing antibodies remained inactive when tested on primary HIV-1 isolates, casting doubts on the efficacy of gp120-based vaccines in the natural setting.

Can J Public Health 1996 May-Jun;87 Suppl 1:S11-4, S11-5 HIV/AIDS in the context of culture: selection of ethnocultural communities for study in Canada. [Article in English, French] Cappon P, Adrien A, Godin G, Singer SM, Maticka-Tyndale E, Willms DG, Daus T. Laurentian University, Sudbury, ON. This article reports on the methodology used to select six ethnocultural communities invited to participate in subsequent phases of the project on HIV/AIDS in the context of culture in Canada. Selection was based on quantitative data on demography, qualitative assessment of ethnocultural cohesion; and quantitative data and qualitative data of exposure to risk for sexually transmitted disease. A principle of partnership insured that the final selection was completed by interaction between the investigators and the National Advisory Committee representing ethnocultural communities in Canada.

Cancer Treat Res 2001;104:1-18 Epidemiology of HIV-associated malignancies. Dal Maso L, Serraino D, Franceschi S. Servizio di Epidemiologia, Centro di Riferimento Oncologico & Servizio di Epidemiologia delle Malattie Infettive, I.R.C.C.S. Lazzaro

Spallanzani.

Cell Mol Biol (Noisy-le-grand) 1995 May;41(3):345-50 Pending problem of "silent" human immunodeficiency virus infection. Bentwich Z, Bar-Yehuda S, Nagai K, Wainberg MA, Kalinkovich A, Jehuda-Cohen T. Ruth Ben Ari Institute of Clinical Immunology, Kaplan Hospital, Hebrew University Medical School, Rehovot, Israel. The problem of "silent" HIV infection is reviewed. Overall, the number of proven "silent" infection in several at-risk populations, including HIV exposed health-care workers, homosexuals, IV drug addicts and children born to HIV-infected mothers, has been very low. Contrary to these observations, we describe a very high prevalence of HIV specific immunity and positive HIV specific PCR signals in an Ethiopian immigrant population recently arrived in Israel.

Cent Afr J Med 1996 Mar;42(3):80-5 Reproductive and sexual health: a research and developmental challenge. Mbizvo MT. Department of Obstetrics and Gynaecology, University of Zimbabwe, Harare, Zimbabwe. There is a growing awareness of the burden and implications of reproductive ill health as contributed by unsafe motherhood (during pregnancy, childbirth, abortion), reproductive tract infection (RTIs) and cancer, sexually transmitted infections (STIs) including the human immunodeficiency virus (HIV), poorly regulated fertility, infertility, unwanted pregnancy and adolescent/teenage sexuality and pregnancy. Sexual health further entails a state of well-being in expression of sexuality, prevention of unwanted pregnancies, prevention of STIs and AIDS and freedom from sexual abuse and violence. Reproductive health is increasingly being recognized as one of the corner stones of health and a major determinant and indicator of human social development.

Cent Afr J Med 1997 Nov;43(11):334-9 Tuberculosis and iron overload in Africa: a review. Moyo VM, Gangaidzo IT, Gordeuk VR, Kiire CF, Macphail AP. Department of Medicine, University of Zimbabwe Medical School, Avondale, Harare, Zimbabwe. Both pulmonary tuberculosis and dietary iron overload are common conditions in sub-Saharan Africa. The incidence of tuberculosis has increased markedly over the last decade, primarily as a result of the rapid spread of infection with the human immunodeficiency virus (HIV). It is possible that the prevention and treatment of dietary iron overload could contribute to the control of tuberculosis in African populations.

Chem Immunol 1993;56:61-77 Antigenic and immunogenic sites of HIV-2 glycoproteins. Chiodi F, Bjorling E, Samuelsson A, Norrby E. Department of Virology, Karolinska Institute, Stockholm, Sweden.

Ciba Found Symp 1993;175:197-212; discussion 212-4 Reproductive health, population growth, economic development and environmental change. Lincoln DW. MRC Reproductive Biology Unit, University of Edinburgh Centre for Reproductive Biology, UK. World population will increase by 1000 million, or by 20%, within 10 years. Ninety-five per cent of this increase will occur in the South, in areas that are already economically, environmentally and politically fragile. Morbidity and mortality associated with reproduction will be greater in the current decade than in any period in human history. Annually, 40-60 million pregnancies will be terminated and 5-10 million children will die within one year of birth. AIDS-related infections, e.g. tuberculosis, will undermine health care in Africa (and elsewhere) and in places AIDS-related deaths will decimate the work-force.

Clin Exp Dermatol 1994 Jul;19(4):335-40 Hairy leucoplakia and HIV-2--a case report and review of the literature. Labandeira J, Peteiro C, Toribio J. Department of Dermatology, General Hospital of Galicia, Faculty of Medicine, Santiago de Compostela, Spain. Type 2 human immunodeficiency virus (HIV-2), originally confined to West Africa, has lately appeared with increasing frequency in Europe. Oral lesions affect a large proportion of patients with AIDS. Hairy leucoplakia (HL), a clinical expression of Epstein-Barr virus (EBV), is a lesion of the oral mucosa (usually the lateral margin of the tongue) that is observed in patients who are immunocompromised due to HIV or, more rarely, due to immunosuppressive medication or other causes.

Clin Infect Dis 1993 Nov;17 Suppl 2:S329-36 AIDS in the

developing world: an epidemiologic overview. Berkely S. Health Sciences Division, Rockefeller Foundation, New York, New York 10036. The pandemic of human immunodeficiency virus (HIV) infection is rapidly becoming a tropical disease. Sub-Saharan Africa alone currently accounts for approximately 60% of the estimated > 11 million infections worldwide. In Africs the virus is transmitted heterosexually and in many areas is now widely dispersed in the general population. Spread of HIV in Asia has been more recent, with current estimates of 2 million infections, but has been very rapid in South and Southeast Asia. With this rapid spread of the infection, there may be as many as 26 million infections--most in developing countries--by the year 2000.

Clin Lab Med 1996 Sep;16(3):697-716 Tuberculosis bacteriology laboratory services and incremental protocols for developing countries. Laszlo A. National Reference Center for Tuberculosis, Laboratory Center for Disease Control, Health Canada, Ottawa, Ontario, Canada. Tuberculosis causes more deaths worldwide than any other single infectious disease.

Most new cases occur in developing countries, where the emergence of HIV/AIDS-associated multidrug-resistant Mycobacterium tuberculosis could disrupt the effective delivery of chemotherapy. Diagnosis, one of the cornerstones of the modern national tuberculosis control programs in developing countries, is based on sputum smear microscopy, which can be delivered effectively only through a national laboratory network.

Clin Microbiol Rev 2001 Apr;14(2):327-35 Global impact of human immunodeficiency virus and AIDS. Gayle HD, Hill GL. National Center for HIV, STD, and TB Prevention, Centers for Disease Control and Prevention, Atlanta, Georgia 30333, USA. This review provides information on the epidemiology, economic impact, and intervention strategies for the human immunodeficiency virus (HIV)/AIDS pandemic in developing countries. According to the World Health Organization and the Joint United Nations Programme on HIV/AIDS (UNAIDS) at the end of 1999, an estimated 34.3 million people were living with HIV/AIDS. Most of the people living with HIV, 95% of the global total, live in developing countries. Examples of the impact of HIV/AIDS in Africa, Asia, Latin America, the Caribbean, and the Newly Independent States provide insight into the demographics, modes of exposure, treatment and prevention options, and the economic effect of the epidemic on the global community.

Clin Perinatol 1994 Mar;21(1):1-14 The growing impact of the HIV/AIDS pandemic on children born to HIV-infected women. Chin J. School of Public Health, Department of BioMedical and Environmental Sciences, University of California, Berkeley. The increasing numbers of children born to HIV-infected women poses formidable problems for maternal and child health programs throughout the world. Between 20% and 40% of these children will be infected with HIV and most are expected to die by the age of 5 years as a result. The vast majority of the uninfected children will be orphaned before age 15 years as their mothers and fathers die of AIDS.

Clin Podiatr Med Surg 1998 Apr;15(2):179-87 Epidemiology of HIV and AIDS. A retrospective look. Signorelli D, Joseph RJ 2nd. Ocean Regional Surgical Podiatric Group, Santa Ana, California, USA. This retrospective look at literature and information regarding the epidemiology of HIV and its progression to AIDS is based on many worldwide sources to determine with some certainty the true severity of the epidemic. The purpose of this article is to permit the reader to become more informed concerning the epidemic, based on a global outlook.

Commun Dis Public Health 1999 Jun;2(2):85-95 The global impact of HIV infection and disease. Nicoll A, Gill ON. HIV and STD Division, PHLS Communicable Disease Surveillance Centre, London. anicoll@phls.co.uk Patterns of HIV infection and disease are changing. HIV will soon enter the top five causes of death worldwide and is now believed to cause more deaths than malaria. Commonwealth countries account for around 60% of prevalent HIV infections worldwide. Around half of all global HIV transmissions are to people under 25 years of age. HIV is lowering life expectancy and reversing gains in child survival in east and central

Africa. The incidence and prevalence of HIV infection have increased enormously in southern Africa recently. A more generalised pattern of heterosexual HIV transmission is emerging in parts of South and South East Asia. Surveillance methods need to adapt to changing patterns of infection and disease.

Commun Dis Public Health 2000 Jun;3(2):78-9 Comment in: Commun Dis Public Health. 2000 Dec;3(4):307-8. Science, sense, and nonsense about HIV in Africa. Nicoll A, Killewo J.

Curationis 1993 Jun;16(2):11-6 AIDS: problems encountered in anthropological research. Boulogne G.

Curr Opin Immunol 2001 Oct;13(5):523-7 The state of immunology in Africa: HIV/AIDS and malaria. Leke RG. HIV and malaria are two major infections that are responsible for the greatest burden of diseases, morbidity and mortality in the African population. Successful research has been undertaken in Africa into novel means of monitoring HIV disease progression and in identifying vaccine candidates.

Curr Opin Oncol 1992 Aug;4(4):667-73 Erratum in: Curr Opin Oncol 1992 Oct;4(5):999 Kaposi's sarcoma. Cho J, Chachoua A. New York University Medical Center, New York. In the era before the acquired immunodeficiency syndrome, Kaposi's sarcoma was a rare cutaneous event. Most reported cases usually originated from one of two geographic regions, an induced immunosuppressed state, or sporadically with various neoplasms that have been known to cause immunosuppression.

Curr Opin Oncol 1995 Sep;7(5):450-5 An integrated approach to the epidemiology of Kaposi's sarcoma. Jacobson LP, Armenian HK. School of Hygiene and Public Health, Johns Hopkins University, Baltimore, MD 21205, USA. As an AIDS-defining illness, Kaposi's sarcoma primarily occurs among HIV-infected homosexual men in developed countries and among men and women in Africa. Except in Africa, Kaposi's sarcoma was rarely diagnosed prior to the AIDS epidemic. The clustering of cases geographically and by gender suggest an environmental influence. Epidemiologic evidence of an infectious cofactor for the disease is presented with the recent findings of herpetic-like viral DNA in Kaposi's sarcoma tissue.

Curr Opin Pulm Med 2000 May;6(3):174-9 Dynamics and control of the global tuberculosis epidemic. Bleed D, Dye C, Raviglione MC. Communicable Diseases, World Health Organization, Geneva, Switzerland. Studies of disease burden have reaffirmed that tuberculosis is among the top 10 causes of death in the world. The tuberculosis epidemic in most countries could eventually be brought under control by implementing the World Health Organization's (WHO) directly observed therapy, short course (DOTS) strategy, although tuberculosis linked to human immunodeficiency virus (HIV) in Africa and multidrug-resistant tuberculosis (MDR-TB) in the former Soviet Union urgently demand adaptations and extensions of DOTS. Most high-incidence countries have achieved treatment success rates approaching the WHO 85% target in pilot projects.

Curr Opin Pulm Med 2000 May;6(3):180-6 Adult tuberculosis overview: African versus Western perspectives. Johnson JL, Ellner JJ.

Department of Medicine, Case Western Reserve University and University Hospitals of Cleveland, Ohio 44106-4984, USA. jlj@po.cwru.edu Tuberculosis is currently an enormous global health problem. In industrialized countries in Western Europe and North America, tuberculosis case rates are low and an increasing proportion of cases now occur in foreign-born individuals and in marginalized populations, including the homeless, prisoners, drug users, and persons with human immunodeficiency virus (HIV) infection or acquired immunodeficiency syndrome (AIDS). In contrast, the burden of tuberculosis in sub-Saharan Africa continues to grow, largely fueled by the HIV pandemic and poor public health infrastructure.

Curr Opin Rheumatol 2000 Jul;12(4):281-6 Spondyloarthropathies in sub-Saharan Africa. Mijiyawa M, Oniankitan O, Khan MA. Service de Rhumatologie, CHU-Tokoin de Lome, Togo. mijiyawa@syfed.tg.refer.org HLA-B27 is virtually absent in most of the sub-Saharan Africa populations, and ankylosing spondylitis is rare; only a few patients have been reported from central and southern Africa. HLA-B27 was present in only one of 17 patients (6%). The disease shows clinical features that are similar to those observed in white HLA-B27-negative patients with ankylosing spondylitis; ie, the disease onset is later compared with HLAB27-positive patients, the patients rarely get acute anterior uveitis as one of the extra-articular manifestations, and familial occurrence of ankylosing spondylitis is rarely observed. There is a virtual absence of ankylosing spondylitis even in the west African countries of Gambia and Senegal, where 3% to 6% of the general population has HLA-B27. The epidemic of HIV infection in sub-Saharan Africa in recent years, however, has been associated with a dramatic upsurge in the prevalence of spondyloarthropathies other than ankylosing spondylitis, primarily reactive arthritis and undifferentiated forms of the disease, and less often psoriatic arthritis. HLA-B27, because of its rarity and virtual lack of association with the observed cases of spondyloarthropathy in this population, cannot be used as an aid to diagnosis of spondyloarthropathy in black Africans.

Dermatol Clin 1995 Jul;13(3):505-23 Epidemiology of the leishmaniases. Magill AJ. Department of Immunology, Walter Reed Army Institute of Research, Washington, D.C., USA. The leishmaniases are a group of zoonotic infections caused by protozoan parasites of the genus Leishmania. These infections produce a variety of different clinical diseases depending on the virulence or tropism of the parasite and differential host immune responses. Newly recognized clinical presentations, such as viscerotropic leishmaniasis in American military veterans of Operation Desert Storm, continue to challenge clinicians. Epidemics of classic visceral leishmaniasis leading to thousands of deaths are ongoing in Brazil, India, and the Sudan. Epidemics of localized cutaneous leishmaniasis are ongoing in many areas of South America, North Africa, and Central Asia.

Diagn Microbiol Infect Dis 1999 Jun;34(2):139-46 The return of tuberculosis. Fatkenheuer G, Taelman H, Lepage P, Schwenk A, Wenzel R. Department I of Internal Medicine, University of Koln, Germany. At the end of the 20th century, tuberculosis remains a major public health issue. In developing countries tuberculosis is a leading cause of morbidity and mortality, and the spread of the HIV epidemic contributes significantly to the worsening of the situation. Coinfection with tuberculosis and HIV results in special diagnostic and therapeutic problems and uses up larger amounts of medical resources in developing countries. Outbreaks of multidrug resistant tuberculosis (MDR-TB) were first reported from US-American centers caring for HIV patients, but have now been observed in many other countries.

Dis Mon 1998 Oct;44(10):545-606 Human immunodeficiency virus infection, Part I. Horowitz HW, Telzak EE, Sepkowitz KA, Wormser GP. Department of Medicine, New York Medical College, Valhalla, USA. Initially recognized in 1982, acquired immunodeficiency syndrome (AIDS) has been the leading cause of death among young adults in the United States for much of this decade, and it has had a devastating impact on people in the developing world. It is estimated that 42 million people worldwide have been infected with human immunodeficiency virus (HIV), the virus that causes AIDS, and that almost 12 million people have died from AIDS-related diseases through 1997. Among these 12 million are 3 million children.

Drug Saf 1995 Apr;12(4):274-82 A risk-benefit assessment of zidovudine in the prevention of perinatal HIV transmission. Newell ML, Gibb DM. Unit of Epidemiology and Biostatistics, Institute of Child Health, London, England. Mother-to-child transmission is the main mode of acquisition of HIV infection for children, and the estimated rate of vertical transmission ranges from 15 to 20% in Europe, 15 to 25% in the US and 25 to 35% in Africa. Vertical transmission is associated with clinical and immunological progression of disease in the mother, breastfeeding and possibly with vaginal delivery. Recently, the findings of the American/French AIDS Clinical Trial Group (ACTG) trial 076 showed that in women with mildly symptomatic HIV disease and no prior treatment with antiretroviral drugs during the pregnancy, zidovudine (ZDV, 3'-azido-3'-deoxythymidine, AZT) reduced the risk of vertical transmission when administered during pregnancy and delivery and to the infant in the first 6 weeks of life. No significant adverse effects were observed in either the mothers or neonates. Further trials with different zidovudine regimens and other strategies to prevent vertical transmission are being planned in several countries.

Early Hum Dev 2000 Apr;58(1):1-16 Epidemiology of HIV infection in the newborn. Thorne C, Newell ML. Institute of Child Health, Department of Pediatric Epidemiology, 30 Guildford Street, London, UK. Vertical transmission of HIV infection can take place in utero, during delivery and postnatally through breastfeeding, with about three-quarters of infections occurring around the time of delivery in non-breastfeeding populations. In Europe, in the absence of specific interventions, the vertical transmission rate was 15-20%. High maternal load is the major risk factor for both intra-uterine and intra-partum mother-to-child transmission. Prematurity is the most common adverse neonatal outcome associated with maternal HIV infection. Earlier diagnosis of pediatric HIV infection than previously available is now possible with virological tests, particularly HIV DNA polymerase chain reaction.

East Afr Med J 1994 Nov;71(11):736-8 Absence of neutropenia in African patients with AIDS and associated pyomyositis. Ansaloni L, Acaye GL. Ambrosoli Memorial Hospital, Kalongo, Kitgum District, Uganda. The association between AIDS and pyomyositis was recently pointed out in temperate and tropical countries. In Western countries, the patients affected by pyomyositis associated with AIDS in most cases are neutropenic. We compare a group of 17 patients with pyomyositis and AIDS living in temperate climates from the literature, and 11 patients affected by the same association seen by us in northern Uganda. The patients from Western countries were significantly more neutropenic and their mean of the neutrophil count was significantly lower when compared with our group. We suggest that the defective neutrophil function associated with HIV infection play a major role in the pathogenesis of pyomyositis in our patients.

East Afr Med J 1995 Jan;72(1):64-8 Pneumocystis carinii: a review. Mpfizi BI, Kamamfu G, Muhirwa G, Floch JJ, Aubry P. Institute of Public Health,

Makerere University, Kampala, Uganda. Pneumocystis carinii has been increasingly recognized as an important cause of opportunistic infection in immune-deficient hosts. The prevalence of pneumocystis pneumonia (PCP) in Africa used to be neglected and underestimated due to difficult methods of isolating the infection. In this review, the authors discuss the nature of the parasite, and methods of diagnosis.

East Afr Med J 1996 Jan;73(1):13-9
Human immunodeficiency virus infection and AIDS in east Africa: challenges and possibilities for prevention and control. Mhalu FS, Lyamuya E. Department of Microbiology/Immunology, Muhimbili University College of Health Sciences, Dar es Salaam, Tanzania. Human immunodeficiency infection and AIDS are a major recent microbial infection in east Africa with serious health and socioeconomic impacts in the region. At present HIV infection and AIDS account for more than 50% of adult medical admissions into some of the national and provincial hospitals as well as for 10-15% of pediatric admissions. AIDS is also at present the commonest

cause of death among those aged 15-45 years. Tuberculosis, a closely associated disease to HIV infection, has increased more than three fold in some countries in the region. While knowledge and tools for preventing HIV transmission are available in the world, prospects for AIDS control in east Africa appear gloomy unless major efforts are made in the reduction of poverty, ignorance and in the control of other common sexually transmitted diseases.

East Afr Med J 1996 Jan;73(1):20-6
Human immunodeficiency virus and AIDS in Uganda. Mugerwa RD, Marum LH, Serwadda D. Department of Medicine, Makerere University Medical School, Kampala, Uganda. HIV-1 infection, initially described as "slim disease", was first recognized in Uganda in 1982, and is now a predominant health problem. Approximately 1.5 million Ugandans are now infected, largely through heterosexual transmission. In many areas half of adult deaths are now caused by HIV. Seroprevalence rates in urban antenatal clinics have been dropping in the last several years, as have rates in young adults in two rural community cohorts where the epidemic is long established. Tuberculosis

cases and admissions have increased dramatically.

East Afr Med J 1996 May;73(5 Suppl):S29-30 Effect of HIV infection on the incidence of lymphoma in Africa. Lucas SB, De Cock KM, Peacock C, Diomande M, Kadio A. Dept of Histopathology, UCL Medical School, London.

East Afr Med J 1997 Dec;74(12):772-6 Socio-cultural and economic aspects of AIDS in Uganda: a review. Monk F, Ineichen B. Imperial College of Science Technology and Medicine, London. AIDS is long-established in Uganda; prevalence rates are high. Most transmission is by heterosexual intercourse, and has been associated with population movements, especially of traders. Treatment resources are very limited and expensive. Some sexual practices inhibit contraceptive use. Attitudes towards AIDS and its testing reveal contradictions, although contraceptive knowledge is widespread. Folk beliefs have not been studied. Government guidelines have beenproduced, although these do not inform clinical attitudes. Indications suggest that prevalence in the long-term may be decreasing.

East Afr Med J 1997 Jun;74(6):341-2 Comment on: East Afr Med J. 1997 Jun;74(6):343-7. Long distance truck driving: its role in the dynamics of HIV/AIDS epidemic. McLigeyo SO.

East Afr Med J 1998 Jun;75(6):358-63 Contemporary treatment of tuberculosis in HIV prevalent countries in sub-Saharan Africa. Nuwaha F. Department of Community Health, Mbarara University, Uganda. The HIV pandemic has been worst felt in sub-Saharan Africa. Tuberculosis is an opportunistic disease in the course of HIV infection and in the region, where the prevalence of both M. tuberculosis and HIV are very high, tuberculosis has become a major complication of HIV infection. The annual risk of tuberculosis infection remains high (1.5 to 2.5%) which is more than fifty times compared to the rates in Western Europe and the prevalence of HIV infection in tuberculosis patients ranges between 18 to 67%. More than 35% of the cases in most countries of sub-Saharan Africa are attributed to HIV.

East Afr Med J 1998 Sep;75(9):520-7 Chemoprophylaxis for tuberculosis in HIV-infected individuals in sub-Saharan Africa. Nuwaha F. Department of Community Health, Mbarara University, Uganda. OBJECTIVE: To examine the role of chemoprophylaxis as a public health strategy for the control of tuberculosis in sub-Saharan Africa. DATA CONCLUSIONS: Because chemoprophylaxis for HIV associated TB makes economic and epidemiological sense, large national programmes should be initiated in sub-Saharan Africa. Operational research is necessary to define the best ways to deliver chemoprophylaxis to the majority of the HIV infected persons and to test the cost-effectiveness of chemoprophylaxis in established national programmes.

Emerg Infect Dis 2001 Nov-Dec;7(6):927-32 Trichomonas vaginalis, HIV, and African-Americans. Sorvillo F, Smith L, Kerndt P, Ash L. Department of Epidemiology, School of Public Health, University of California, Los Angeles, 90024, USA. fsorviill@ucla.edu Trichomonas vaginalis may be emerging as one of the most important cofactors in amplifying HIV transmission, particularly in African-American communities of the United States. In a person co-infected with HIV, the pathology induced by T. vaginalis infection can increase HIV shedding. Trichomonas infection may also act to expand the portal of entry for HIV in an HIV-negative person. Studies from Africa have suggested that T. vaginalis infection may increase the rate of HIV transmission by approximately twofold. Available data indicate that T. vaginalis is highly prevalent among African-Americans in major urban centers of the United States and is often the most common sexually transmitted infection in black women. Even if T. vaginalis increases the risk of HIV transmission by a small amount, this could translate into an important amplifying effect since Trichomonas is so common. Substantial HIV transmission may be attributable to T. vaginalis in African-American communities of the United States.

Emerg Med Clin North Am 1995 Feb;13(1):1-25 The epidemiology of the acquired immunodeficiency syndrome in the 1990s. Quinn TC. Division of Infectious Diseases, Johns Hopkins University School of Medicine. Since the recognition of AIDS in 1981, it has become a global pandemic afflicting more than 6 million people worldwide. To date, more than

22 million people are infected with HIV-1, the cause of AIDS, and more than 40 million people may be infected with HIV by the year 2000. In the United States, AIDS has become the leading cause of death in young men and the fourth leading cause of death in young women. HIV is primarily transmitted sexually, parenterally, and perinatally, with increasing evidence of heterosexual transmission in the United States and worldwide. Factors associated with transmission and susceptibility to HIV are discussed, and the natural history of HIV and means of intervention are detailed in this article.

Epidemiol Rev 1994;16(2):403-17 Surveillance of acquired immunodeficiency syndrome in Africa. An analysis of evaluations of the World Health Organization and other clinical definitions. Belec L, Brogan T, Mbopi Keou FX, Georges AJ. Department of Microbiology (Virology), Broussais University Hospital, Paris, France.

Epidemiology 1993 Jan;4(1):63-72 AIDS in sub-Saharan Africa: the epidemiology of heterosexual transmission and the prospects for prevention. Hunter DJ. Department of Epidemiology,

Harvard School of Public Health, Boston, MA 02115. As the epidemic of the acquired immunodeficiency syndrome (AIDS) in sub-Saharan Africa enters its second decade, much has been learned about the distribution and determinants of the disease and its causative agent, the human immunodeficiency virus (HIV). Over 6 million people, or 2.5% of the adult population, are thought to be infected with HIV. The distribution of HIV is largely determined by sexual behavior; as for other sexually transmitted diseases, the characteristics of sexual networks determine the extent and rate of spread of HIV. Female sex workers and their male clients are at high risk for HIV and have been important in initiating the epidemic in many African countries.

Ethiop Med J 2000 Oct;38(4):283-302 The HIV epidemic and the state of its surveillance in Ethiopia. Kebede D, Aklilu M, Sanders E. Department of Community Health, Faculty of Medicine, Addis Ababa University, P.O.Box 31048, Addis Ababa. A review of the information on the HIV epidemic in Ethiopia is important to guide policy and action. Published and unpublished reports and surveillance data from records of governmental and non-governmental institutions were examined to assess the extent of the epidemic. It appears that the HIV/AIDS epidemic has affected a large segment of the urban population. Surveillance data from pregnant women attending antenatal clinics indicate a decreasing trend in the prevalence of HIV in Addis Ababa. Similarly, data from blood donors from the majority of transfusion centres in the country indicate a decrease in prevalence. However, further studies will be required to establish the validity of these findings. Currently available data are not adequate to accurately measure the level of infection in rural areas where 85% of the population live.

Eur J Cancer 2001 Jul;37(10):1188-201 Epidemiology of AIDS-related tumours in developed and developing countries. Dal Maso L, Serraino D, Franceschi S. Servizio di Epidemiologia, Centro di Riferimento Oncologico, IRCCS, Istituto Nazionale Tumori, Via Pedemontana Occ., 33081 (PN), Aviano, Italy. epidemiology@cro.it AIDS-associated illnesses include Kaposi's sarcoma (KS), non-Hodgkin's lymphoma (NHL), and, since 1993, invasive cervical cancer (ICC). Between 1988 and 1998, among AIDS cases reported in western Europe, 9.6% had KS and 3.9% had NHL as AIDS-defining illnesses. Between 1988 and 1998, the frequency of KS decreased from 13.4 to 6.4%, while NHL increased from 3.8 to 5.3%. Estimates of the relative risk (RR) of neoplasms in HIV-seropositive populations came from population-based cancer and AIDS registries linkage studies conducted in the United States, Italy and Australia and from a few cohort and case-control studies. In adults with HIV/AIDS, the RR was over 1000 for KS and ranged between 14 for low-grade NHL and over 300 for high-grade NHL. For Hodgkin's disease (HD), a consistent 10-fold higher RR was observed. For cervical and other anogenital tumours associated with human papilloma virus, risk increases were 2- and 12-fold, depending upon location. In Africa, the AIDS epidemic led to KS becoming the most common cancer type in men in several areas. The RR of AIDS-associated tumours were lower in Africa than those reported in western countries.

Eur J Med Res 1999 Aug 25;4(8):341-4 HIV and AIDS in Africa: impact on mother and child health. Van de Perre P. Centre Muraz, Organisation de Coordination et de Cooperation pour la lutte contre les Grandes Endemies (OCCGE), 01 BP 153, Bobo-Dioulasso, Burkina Faso. direction.muraz@fasonet.bf
Mother to child transmission of HIV-1 is a leading challenge of public health in developing countries. Various risk factors for vertical transmission of HIV have been identified, and both prenatal and postnatal infection by breast feeding occur. A bundle of interventions has lead to a dramatic drop of infection rates in industrialised countries. For the developing countries it is crucial to increase accessibility of health services, to perform prevention campaigns, and to provide antiretroviral prophylaxis for pregnant women.

Eur J Obstet Gynecol Reprod Biol 1996 Oct;69(1):41-5 Comment in: Eur J Obstet Gynecol Reprod Biol. 1996 Oct;69(1):3-4. Primary reproductive health care in Tanzania. Walraven GE. Sumve Designated District Hospital, Mantare via Mwanza, Tanzania.
The introduction of community based reproductive health care programmes in Tanzania integrated within primary health care (PHC) programmes is discussed. These programmes should address safe motherhood, fertility awareness and sexually transmitted diseases (STDs), including AIDS. It is argued that the proposed primary reproductive health care programmes will only be sustainable if community participation is achieved, and if combined with improved woman and child health programmes. Sensitized communities, who have learned how to prioritize the problems identified and the appropriate actions to take, will have to be linked at the local level with well trained and supervised health workers, having proper equipment and supplies.

Eur J Pediatr Surg 1998 Feb;8(1):47-51 Cancrum oris (noma) in children. Valadas G, Leal MJ. Servico de Cirurgia Pediatrica, Hospital Dona Estefania, Lisboa, Portugal.
Cancrum oris, noma or gangrenous stomatitis is a disease which affects primarily undernourished and immunosuppressed young children. Frequent in underdeveloped countries, it also is seen in rare cases of patients with AIDS and

leukemia in America and in Europe. Once fatal, the disease is now better understood and today the repair of its terrible sequels is looked upon as a great surgical challenge. This paper reports a case of noma in a 3-year-old black African female admitted to this Service.

Genetica 1995;95(1-3):173-93 The epidemiology and transmission of AIDS: a hypothesis linking behavioural and biological determinants to time, person and place. Stewart GT. Emeritus Professor of Public Health, University of Glasgow, UK. Epidemiologically, the Acquired Immune Deficiency Syndrome, AIDS, is transmitted and distributed in the USA and Europe almost entirely in well-defined subsets of populations engaging in, or subjected to, the effects of behaviours which carry high risks of genital and systemic infections. The persons predominantly affected are those engaging in promiscuous homosexual and bisexual activity, regular use of addictive drugs, and their sexual and recreational partners. In such persons and in subsets of populations with corresponding life-styles, the risk of AIDS increases by orders of magnitude. Because of continuity of risk behaviour and

of associated indicator infections, the incidence of AIDS over 3-5 year periods is predictable to within 10% of actual totals of registered cases in the USA and UK.

Genitourin Med 1993 Aug;69(4):297-300 Soap and water prophylaxis for limiting genital ulcer disease and HIV-1 infection in men in sub-Saharan Africa. O'Farrell N. Department of Genito-urinary Medicine, Guy's Hospitals, London, UK. In general, East, Central and Southern Africa appear to be worse affected by HIV-1 infection than West Africa. So far there is little evidence to suggest that differences in either sexual behaviour or numbers of sexual partners could account for this disparity. Two risk factors in men for acquiring HIV-1, that tend to vary along this geographical divide, are lack of circumcision and genital ulcer disease (GUD) which are much less common in West Africa. Although uncircumcised men with GUD are an important high frequency HIV-1 transmitter core group, few interventions have targeted such individuals. Given the recent expansion in AIDS-related technologies, is it possible that methods effective in limiting GUD in the preantibiotic era have been overlooked? During the first and second world wars, chancroid, the commonest cause of GUD in Africa today, was controlled successfully with various prophylactics including soap and water. Many parts of Africa are undergoing social upheaval against a background of violence, and in this environment soap and water prophylaxis would now seem to merit re-evaluation as an intervention for preventing both GUD and HIV-1 in uncircumcised men.

Genitourin Med 1994 Dec;70(6):394-8 Comment in: Genitourin Med. 1995 Apr;71(2):136. Kaposi's sarcoma in HIV infected women in Germany: more evidence for sexual transmission. A report of 10 cases and review of the literature. Albrecht H, Helm EB, Plettenberg A, Emminger C, Heise W, Schwartlander B, Stellbrink HJ. Department of Internal Medicine, University Clinic Eppendorf, Hamburg. OBJECTIVE--To assess the natural history of Kaposi's sarcoma (KS) in HIV-positive women living in Germany. METHODS--All physicians reporting the diagnosis of KS in a female patient were contacted and asked for detailed information. DESIGN--

Descriptive study of clinical, epidemiological and immunological data of ten women with biopsy-proven KS living in Germany were evaluated. The results are compared with those of other previously published studies of women with KS from Italy, France and the USA. CONCLUSIONS--KS seems to run a particularly aggressive course in women. Our data are consistent with a sexually transmittable aetiological agent of KS. Prostitution, an issue yet to be addressed by other authors reporting series of women with KS, was reported in four of our patients. Further studies are needed to clarify the significance of this finding.

Genitourin Med 1995 Feb;71(1):27-31 Global eradication of donovanosis: an opportunity for limiting the spread of HIV-1 infection. O'Farrell N. Department of Genitourinary Medicine, Guy's Hospital, London, UK. Genital ulcer disease (GUD) is well recognised in the developing world as a co-factor for heterosexual HIV transmission. Men with GUD are an important high frequency HIV transmitter core group in the general population but few interventions have targeted such individuals so far. Donovanosis is an uncommon GUD with low infectivity characterised by large ulcers that bleed readily and has been identified as a risk factor for HIV in men in Durban, South Africa. Donovanosis is also endemic in Papua New Guinea, India, Brazil and amongst the Aboriginal community in Australia. This curious geographical distribution is unique to any of the sexually transmitted diseases (STD) and might lend itself to control measures not tried previously.

Health Transit Rev 1993;3(Suppl):1-16 African families and AIDS: context, reactions and potential interventions. Caldwell J, Caldwell P, Ankrah EM, Anarfi JK, Agyeman DK, Awusabo-Asare K, Orubuloye IO. Health Transition Centre, NCEPH, ANU, Canberra, Australia. This paper reviews publications and research reports on how sub-Saharan African families have been affected by, and reacted to, the AIDS epidemic. The nature of the African family and its variation across the regions is shown to be basic to both an understanding of how the epidemic spread and of its impact. The volume of good social science research

undertaken until now on the disease in Africa is shown to be extremely small relative to the need.

Health Transit Rev 1995;5 Suppl:1-26 Social context of HIV infection in Uganda. Adeokun LA, Twa-Twa J, Ssekiboobo A, Nalwadda R. Institute of Statistics and Applied Economics, Makerere University, Kampala, Uganda. Some of the important policy and research implications of accumulating HIV/AIDS data are being ignored because of the attraction of social science research focused on the "multiple sexual mechanism' of infection and transmission. Attention is drawn to the other policy and research issues relating to information on the timing of infection through a reanalysis of existing data on cumulative AIDS cases. The most urgent need is to supplement the mainstream research on risk groups with studies of the timing and circumstances of entry into sexual activity in the pre-teen years.

Health Transit Rev 1995;5 Suppl:179-89 The effects of HIV and AIDS on fertility in East and Central Africa. Setel P. National Centre for

Epidemiology and Population Health, Australian National University. Concern has been expressed about the fertility of people infected with HIV: the worry has been that on learning of their condition, HIV-affected individuals may attempt to accomplish unmet reproductive goals knowing that they will not live a normal life span. This article addresses the potential effects of AIDS on fertility and reproductive decisions in East and Central Africa. The problem is seen in terms of a tightly knit continuum of biological, epidemiologic and cultural contexts, and the prevailing conditions of response to the epidemic. AIDS can influence fertility among individuals and groups regardless of any awareness of serostatus by increasing death rates among reproductive populations, and damaging the physical capacities of infected men and women to reproduce. In much of the region, high prevalence of STDs may simultaneously impair the fertility of men and women and increase their risk of contracting HIV.

HIV Clin Trials 2001 Jul-Aug;2(4):356-65 Tuberculosis and HIV infection: epidemiology, immunology, and treatment. Schluger NW, Burzynski J. The Division of Pulmonary, Allergy, and Critical Care Medicine, Columbia University College of Physicians and Surgeons, New York, New York 10032, USA. ns311@columbia.edu Tuberculosis and HIV have combined to present a major threat to global public health. Each disease has a negative effect on the other, and mortality in patients with both tuberculosis and HIV is higher than that caused by either condition alone. In regions such as sub-Saharan Africa, as many as a third or more of all patients with tuberculosis have concomitant HIV infection. In urban centers in developed nations, HIV co-infection may also be quite common.

Hum Pathol 2000 Oct;31(10):1274-98 HIV-1 and its causal relationship to immunosuppression and nervous system disease in AIDS: a review. Sotrel A, Dal Canto MC. Department of Pathology, University of Illinois at Chicago, Chicago, IL, USA. Acquired immune deficiency syndrome (AIDS), caused by human immunodeficiency virus type 1 (HIV-1), has claimed more than 10 million lives over the past 15 years. There are approximately 30 million HIV-positive people worldwide, 89% of whom reside in sub-Saharan Africa and Asia. The intricate relationship between the virus and HIV-related human multisystem pathology prompted scientists to modify many previously established concepts about infectious diseases and immunology, and to test new ones. The results of this work helped resolve many, albeit not all, long-standing problems concerning HIV-1 immune escape, its cellular tropism, and pathogenesis of HIV-related immunosuppression and nervous system disease. The most impressive advances have been made in antiretroviral drug treatment of HIV infection, which has resulted in dramatically reducing AIDS-related mortality, morbidity, and perinatal transmission. However, considering the magnitude of the worldwide HIV-AIDS pandemic, prohibitive cost and unusually exacting nature of combination drug treatment, as well as the emergence of drug-resistant HIV mutants, the disease and virus remain formidable and unpredictable, particularly in the area of prevention and vaccine development.

Immunol Today 1995 Apr;16(4):187-91 Immune activation is a dominant factor in the pathogenesis of African AIDS. Bentwich Z, Kalinkovich A, Weisman Z. R. Ben-Ari Institute of Clinical Immunology, Kaplan Hospital, Hebrew University Hadassah Medical School, Rehovot, Israel. The AIDS epidemic in Africa is very different from the epidemic in the West. As suggested here by Zvi Bentwich, Alexander Kalinkovich and Ziva Weisman, this appears to be primarily a consequence of the over-activation of the immune system in the African population, owing to the extremely high prevalence of infections, particularly helminthic, in Africa. Such activation shifts the cytokine balance towards a T helper 0/2 (Th0/2)-type response, which makes the host more susceptible to infection with human immunodeficiency virus (HIV) and less able to cope with it.

Infect Dis Clin North Am 1998 Mar;12(1):39-46 Group O human immunodeficiency virus-1 infections. Jaffe HW, Schochetman G. Division of AIDS, STD, and TB Laboratory Research, National Center for Infectious Diseases, Centers for Disease Control and Prevention, Atlanta, Georgia, USA. Human immunodeficiency viruses

(HIV), the cause of AIDS, have remarkable genetic diversity. Among the HIV-1 viruses are the "major" (group M) HIV-1 subtypes and genetic "outliers" that have been designated as group O viruses. Group O viruses are most prevalent in parts of Africa, although they have also been reported in Europe and the United States and are associated with AIDS. Because group O viruses are so highly divergent, tests designed to detect group M viruses may be unreliable in the diagnosis of group O infection. Modification of these tests are needed to protect the safety of the blood supply.

Infect Dis Clin North Am 1998 Mar;12(1):63-82 Kaposi's sarcoma and human herpesvirus-8. Greenblatt RM. Infectious Diseases Division, University of California San Francisco, USA. KS is a major cause of morbidity and mortality among AIDS patients and a treatment problem in the sporadic cases that are not associated with HIV. All four forms of the disease are linked to a newly described herpesvirus, HHV-8 or KSHV, via strong epidemiologic associations and biologic plausibility as a causal agent. HHV-8 is also epidemiologically associated with body cavity-based lymphomas, which are almost unique to AIDS, and Castleman's disease. Existing radiation and chemotherapeutic treatments of KS are only partially effective and cause significant adverse effects.

Infection 1999;27 Suppl 2:S39-41 Recent developments in the epidemiology of virus diseases and BSE. Kaaden OR, Truyen U. Institut fur Medizinische Mikrobiologie, Infektions- und Seuchenmedizin, Ludwig-Maximilians-Universitat Munchen and WHO Collaborating Centre for Collection and Evaluation of Data on Comparative Virology, Germany. There is a continuous change in viral epidemics with respect to clinical symptoms, their duration or disappearance and the emergence of new diseases. This can be observed both in human and animal diseases. This evolution of virus diseases is mainly related to three factors: etiological agent, host and environment. As far as genetic alterations of the virus are concerned, two major mechanisms are involved: 1) mutations such as recombination and reassortment; 2) selection for resistance or susceptibility.

Int J Cancer 1999 Nov 12;83(4):481-5 Advances in the epidemiology of HIV-associated non-Hodgkin's lymphoma and other lymphoid neoplasms. Franceschi S, Dal Maso L, La Vecchia C. Servizio di Epidemiologia, Centro di Riferimento Oncologico, Aviano, Italy. epidemiology@ets.it The spectrum of HIV-related lymphoid malignancies certainly includes non-Hodgkin's lymphoma (NHL; i.e., chiefly large-cell lymphoma and Burkitt's lymphoma), primary lymphoma of the brain (PBL) and, possibly, Hodgkin's disease (HD). Since the mid-1990s, several epidemiological studies have led to better quantification of the burden of lymphomas in HIV-infected populations. AIDS surveillance data from 17 western European countries show that between 1988 and 1997 a total of 7,148 AIDS cases had NHL as the AIDS-defining illness. The yearly number of cases rose steadily from 1988 to 1995 but declined thereafter. As a percentage of AIDS-defining illnesses, NHL increased from 3.6% in 1994 to 4.9% in 1997. Percent increases were observed in different strata by area, age group, sex and HIV-transmission group. To estimate relative risk (RR) of NHL and other lymphoid neoplasms in unselected HIV-seropositive populations, records of population-based cancer registries and AIDS registries were linked in the United States, Italy and Australia. RRs for NHL in adults with HIV/AIDS ranged between 14 (for low-grade NHL) to over 300 (for high-grade NHL). For HD, the RR was approximately 10. Limited findings from studies based on death certificates and cohorts of HIV-seropositive persons were consistent with those from registry linkage studies.

Int J Epidemiol 1993 Feb;22(1):127-34 The frontline of HIV1 diffusion in the Central African region: a geographical and epidemiological perspective. Tessier SF, Remy G, Louis JP, Trebucq A. Centre International de l'Enfance, Paris, France. The geographical analysis of the main data on the HIV1 epidemic in Central Africa shows a frontline which has not moved significantly since 1985. The absence of a progressive increase between the countries, demonstrating a discontinuity in space, combined with the observed human and physical continuity within the areas, raises several questions. Are the low-rate areas facing only a simple delay in the diffusion, or is there a real difference between the epidemiological patterns of HIV1 in the two areas? The last hypothesis would impose a revision of the concept of an homogeneous pattern in the epidemiology of HIV1 in Africa. The need for further research is emphasized with the aim of precisely targeting preventive intervention.

Int J Gynaecol Obstet 1994 Feb;44(2):107-12 HIV-1 and reproductive health in Africa. Temmerman M, Chomba EN, Piot P. Department of Medical Microbiology, University of Nairobi, Kenya.

Int J Gynaecol Obstet 1998 Dec;63 Suppl 1:S161-5 HIV: mother to child transmission, current knowledge and on-going studies. Giaquinto C, Ruga E, Giacomet V, Rampon O, D'Elia R. Dipartimento di Pediatria, Padova, Italy. It is estimated that approximately 6000 women of childbearing age, mostly living in the developing world, acquire HIV infection every day. Taking into account that approximately 98% of HIV infected children have acquired HIV from the mother, during pregnancy, at delivery or through breastfeeding, therefore, prevention of mother-to-child transmission (MTCT) is a major health priority.

Int J Infect Dis 2001;5(1):43-8 Systematic review of combination antiretroviral therapy with didanosine plus hydroxyurea: a partial solution to Africa's HIV/AIDS problem? Sanne I, Smego RA Jr, Mendelow BV. Department of Infectious Diseases and Clinical Microbiology, University of Witwaterswand, Johannesburg, Republic of South Africa. Effective antiretroviral therapy remains beyond the reach of most human immunodeficiency virus (HIV)-infected persons living in the third world because of its tremendous cost. The cancer drug, hydroxyurea, inhibits HIV-1 replication in vitro and, when combined with didanosine (ddI), results in significant antiretroviral synergy. In vivo, hydroxyurea specifically targets quiescent lymphocytes and macrophages, important cellular reservoirs for HIV-1, and the combination of ddI plus hydroxyurea effectively reduces plasma HIV-1 RNA levels. Combination ddI-hydroxyurea costs about one-eighth as much as currently recommended triple drug combinations, and several countries in Africa are exploring the feasibility of widescale use of ddI-hydroxyurea for their HIV-infected populations. Intrigued by its potential relevance for Africa, the authors reviewed the literature on the in vitro and clinical efficacy of ddI plus hydroxyurea against HIV.

Int J Occup Environ Health 1998 Oct-Dec;4(4):257-64 Creating alliances for disease management in industrial settings: a case study of HIV/AIDS in workers in South African gold mines. Williams B, Campbell C. London School of Economics and Political Science, U.K. brian@eru.wn.apc.org The epidemic of HIV/AIDS is at an advanced stage in many African countries, but little attention has been given to the impact that this will have in industrial settings. Using the Southern African mining industry as a case study, the authors consider the state of the HIV epidemic and discuss programs that have been undertaken to manage HIV. They critically analyze the reasons current interventions have had little impact on HIV among mine workers, tracing the lack of success to neglect of the social and community contexts within which HIV transmission takes place, as well as the lack of attention to the psychosocial processes and mechanisms underlying disease transmission. Finally, they present an intervention that aims to address the limitations of existing industrial programs and improve the management of sexually transmitted diseases (STDs), including HIV, in a particular occupational setting through creating alliances between a wide range of community stakeholders.

Int J Radiat Oncol Biol Phys 1994 Feb 1;28(3):613-9 Radiation therapy for non-AIDS associated (classic and endemic African) and epidemic Kaposi's sarcoma. Stein ME, Lakier R, Spencer D, Dale J, Kuten A, MacPhail P, Bezwoda WR. Department of Medical Oncology and Hematology, University of the Witwatersrand, Johannesburg, Republic of South Africa. PURPOSE: A retrospective analysis of patients with non-AIDS and AIDS-related Kaposi's sarcoma, who were treated with radiation therapy. CONCLUSION: Radiotherapy is the most useful mode of palliative treatment for all forms of Kaposi's sarcoma in southern African patients.

Int J STD AIDS 1996 Jan-Feb;7(1):4-6 Sexually

transmissible agent and African Kaposi's sarcoma. Matondo P, Sivapalan S. Kaposi's sarcoma (KS) has a higher incidence in some parts of Africa than anywhere else in the world. Recent studies in western homosexual men with AIDS-KS suggest that KS may be caused by a putative sexually transmissible agent. Our analytical review of studies on KS in Africa before and during the AIDS era reveals a disparate epidemiological picture. Its occurrence in sexually inexperienced children; overwhelming male preponderance in an almost exclusively heterosexual population; rarity of concordant couples in areas of very high incidence; sequestration of high incidence to Eastern and Central Africa; and regional variations in incidence even in high-incidence countries are all difficult to reconcile with a conventional sexually transmissible aetiology.

Int J STD AIDS 1996 Jul;7(4):236-43 AIDS in rural Africa: a paradigm for HIV-1 prevention. Hudson CP. Networks of concurrent sexual partnerships may be the primary cause of epidemic spread of HIV-1 in parts of sub-Saharan Africa. This pattern of sexual behaviour increases the likelihood that individuals experiencing primary HIV-1 infection transmit the virus to other persons. Networks of concurrent partnerships are likely to be important in both the early ('epidemic') and late ('endemic') phases of HIV-1 transmission. Interventions should aim to break the sexual networks, whatever the stage of the epidemic.

Int J Tuberc Lung Dis 1998 Oct;2(10):844-51 Comment in: Int J Tuberc Lung Dis. 1999 Dec;3(12):1144. Childhood human immunodeficiency virus and tuberculosis co-infections: reconciling conflicting data. Coovadia HM, Jeena P, Wilkinson D. Department of Paediatrics and Child Health, University of Natal, Durban, South Africa. The impact of the human immunodeficiency virus (HIV) pandemic on childhood tuberculosis (TB) is unclear because of inconsistent and often contradictory findings in different types of studies. We review the evidence which supports or refutes the likelihood that HIV infection in children predisposes them to TB, and conclude that, on balance, HIV during infancy increases the risk of developing TB.

Int J Tuberc Lung Dis 1999 Jun;3(6):457-65 Will DOTS do it? A reappraisal of tuberculosis control in countries with high rates of HIV infection. De Cock KM, Chaisson RE. London School of Hygiene and Tropical Medicine. kmd2@cdc.gov In 1993 the WHO declared tuberculosis a global emergency, and subsequently introduced the DOTS strategy, a technical and management package based on earlier work of the IUATLD and international experience with directly observed therapy. Despite successful implementation of most of the elements of this strategy in several African countries and settings, tuberculosis case rates continue to escalate where the prevalence of HIV infection is high. We explore possible reasons for the failure to control tuberculosis even in the context of tuberculosis programmes that have been considered models for others to emulate.

Int J Tuberc Lung Dis 1999 Jun;3(6):546 HIV-associated mycobacteraemia in West Africa. Bonard D, Aka K, Zahibo JC, You B, Combe P, Anglaret X.

Int J Tuberc Lung Dis 2000 Jul;4(7):606-14 Health sector reform and tuberculosis control: the case of Zambia. Bosman MC. Royal Netherlands Tuberculosis Association, The Hague. bosmanm@who.ch SETTING: Zambia, 1995-1997. OBJECTIVE: To describe the process leading to the collapse of Zambia's National Tuberculosis Programme NTP). CONCLUSIONS: The experience in Zambia demonstrates the urgent need for constructive dialogue between 'health reformers' and 'disease controllers'. The aim of this dialogue would be to develop a model that ensures that tuberculosis patients are properly diagnosed and cured in countries that are embarking on a reform of their health services.

Int J Tuberc Lung Dis 2000 Jul;4(7):627-32 Effective tuberculosis control and health sector reforms in Kenya: challenges of an increasing tuberculosis burden and opportunities through reform. Hanson C, Kibuga D. World Bank, Washington, DC, USA. During the period from 1980 to 1997, the annual number of new tuberculosis cases increased four-fold in Kenya, and had reached approximately 50,000 cases by 1998. During the same time period, the government per capita expenditure on health dropped from US$9.5 to US$3.5. Since 1983, Kenya has been decentralising financial responsibility and decision-making power to the districts. In addition, the late 1980s saw the introduction of cost-sharing schemes for most health services, excluding tuberculosis (TB) treatment. In the midst of these changes, a dual epidemic of TB and HIV/AIDS emerged, and is presently over-burdening the traditional public health system. In response, the National Leprosy and Tuberculosis Control Programme (NLTP) is seeking a wider network of service providers and new approaches to the prevention and treatment of TB in the country.

Int J Tuberc Lung Dis 2001 Jan;5(1):12-23 Pulmonary disease in HIV-infected African children. Graham SM, Coulter JB, Gilks CF. Department of Paediatrics, College of Medicine, University of Malawi. grahamst@sesahs.nsw.gov.au Childhood human immunodeficiency virus (HIV) infection is common in most regions of sub-Saharan Africa. Acute and chronic respiratory diseases are major causes of morbidity and mortality in HIV-infected children. They represent a significant added burden in a region where diagnostic capabilities are limited and management decisions are often made on the basis of clinical guidelines alone. Pneumocystis carinii pneumonia is now recognised as an important cause of acute severe pneumonia and death in HIV-infected infants.

Int Ophthalmol Clin 2000 Spring;40(2):137-52 Infectious causes of uveitis in the developing world. Rathinam SR, Cunningham ET Jr. Uvea Clinic, Aravind Eye Hospital, Madurai, Tamil Nadu, India. Infectious causes of uveitis are common in the developing world and include some causes that are rarely encountered in industrialized nations, such as tuberculosis, leptospirosis, leprosy, onchocerciasis, and cystercicosis. Ocular toxoplasmosis occurs in all countries but is more common in Central and South America, the South Pacific, and western Europe. AIDS-related opportunistic infections occur wherever HIV infection is prevalent, including North and South America, western and eastern Europe, the former Soviet Union, sub-Saharan Africa, and South and Southeast Asia. Physicians who care for patients in the developing world should consider these infectious possibilities whenever their patients develop uveitis.

J Acquir Immune Defic Syndr Hum Retrovirol 1997;14 Suppl 2:S58-67 International HIV and AIDS prevention: Japan/United States collaboration. Umenai T, Narula M, Onuki D, Yamamoto T, Igari T. Department of Health Policy and Planning, School of International Health, University of Tokyo, Japan. As the epicenter of the HIV/AIDS pandemic shifts from Africa to Asia, Japan is becoming ever more aware of the importance of containing and preventing spread of the virus. International collaboration, particularly with the United States, is a logical approach because it allows utilization of expertise from countries in other stages of the pandemic, can prevent duplication of efforts, and complements efforts of the other countries. Further, both Japan and the United States can use their combined influence and prestige to encourage cooperation among all nations.

J Antimicrob Chemother 1996 May;37 Suppl B:113-20 Mycobacteriosis and HIV infection: the new public health challenge. Porter JD. Department of Clinical Sciences, London School of Hygiene and Tropical Medicine, UK. Human immunodeficiency virus (HIV) infection alters the epidemiology of mycobacterial infections. In the industrialised world, this has led to an increase in severe illness associated with Mycobacterium avium-intracellulare complex (MAC) and, in the developing world, to doubling of tuberculosis cases in some countries in Sub-Saharan Africa. The interaction with Mycobacterium tuberculosis occurs when the CD4 count is relatively high (> 200) and tuberculosis (TB) is now the commonest presenting AIDS defining disease in Africa. In international public health terms the interaction between TB and HIV infection has led to the World Health Organisation declaring TB to be a global emergency. Both TB and HIV are diseases of poverty and the key to the reduction of incidence of both diseases is the improvement of socio-economic conditions. Other control methods are case finding and treatment, chemoprophylaxis and BCG vaccination.

J Assoc Nurses AIDS Care 2000 Jul-Aug;11(4):17-26 The sociological spread of HIV/AIDS in South Africa.

Mitton J. South Africa (SA) now accounts for more than 50% of newly reported HIV cases in sub-Saharan Africa annually. In 1993, approximately 90% of those reported as HIV positive in SA were of African descent. This paper examines sociological factors in the spread of HIV in SA through the application of Lalonde's (1974) Health Field Concept. SA's emerging District Health System (DHS) is discussed, as well as barriers to effective implementation and recommendations. Through Lalonde's sociopolitical view of health, a coordinated and multisectorial approach to HIV/AIDS in SA can be established. Without this approach, health care interventions will fail to target the population effectively, thereby reducing effectiveness and sustainability.

J Craniomaxillofac Surg 1994 Apr;22(2):76-80 Oro-facial tumours in Ethiopian patients. Clinical analysis of 108 cases and a review of the literature. Neway M, Eshete S, Minasse M. Department of Oral Maxillofacial Surgery and Dentistry, Yekatit 12 Teaching Hospital, Addis Ababa, Ethiopia. Maxillofacial surgery is a new medical discipline in Ethiopia. Between May 1991 and December 1992, 108 patients with maxillofacial tumours were treated in our Department. These cases are analysed according to their age, sex, anatomical site, histopathological classification of benign and malignant tumours.

J Dermatol 2001 Nov;28(11):617-21 Traveling through skin manifestations of HIV in 2001. Rico MJ. Fujisawa Healthcare, Inc, Deerfield, IL 60066, USA. There are currently over 34 million people worldwide infected with human immunodeficiency virus (HIV) with 15,000 new patients infected each day. The acquired immunodefiency syndrome (AIDS) pandemic has particularly affected the third world and currently over 70% of those infected reside in sub-Saharan Africa. The epicenter of the pandemic is shifting to Asia as HIV infection increases in the densely populated countries of India, China, and SE Asia. Patients with HIV infection develop a variety of mucocutaneous diseases and often present to dermatologists.

J Eukaryot Microbiol 2000 Jan-Feb;47(1):37-9 Leishmania, Trypanosoma and monoxenous trypanosomatids as emerging opportunistic agents. Dedet JP, Pratlong F. Laboratoire de Parasitologie, C.H.U. de Montpellier, 163, France. parasito@sc.univ-montp1.fr Immunosuppression is associated with the occurrence of a large variety of infections, several of them due to opportunistic protozoa. The parasitic protozoa of the family Trypanosomatidae vary greatly in their importance as potential opportunistic pathogens. African trypanosomiasis is no more common nor severe during AIDS. The situation with Chagas' disease, however, is much different. Although the process is not clearly understood, there appears to be a reactivation of Trypanosoma cruzi infection, which can lead to severe meningoencephalitis.

J Infect Chemother 2000 Dec;6(4):196-9 Anti-retroviral treatment in Nigeria: a review. Anyiwo CE, Ifeanyichukwu M. Department of Pathology, Nnamdi Azikiwe University Teaching Hospital, Nnewi, Nigeria. ceanyiwo@Yahoo.com Research studies in Nigeria have been done primarily in the areas of epidemiology, clinical practice, virology, and laboratory diagnosis. Therapy for infection with human immunodeficiency virus (HIV) types 1 and 2 has largely focussed on the treatment of the HIV disease (AIDS) rather than the infection. Therefore, opportunistic infections such as tuberculosis, diarrhea, Herpes zoster, and other skin conditions, and tumors (Kaposi's sarcoma) are essentially the targets for therapy. Two reasons are responsible for the dearth of data on anti-retroviral therapy in Nigeria: there was scepticism about zidovudine, the first anti-retroviral drug to be developed, because of its toxicity, and the subsequent reluctance of the Federal Government to allow it into the country. The other reason was the prohibitive cost, making it impossible for patients to afford.

J Intern Med 2000 Mar;247(3):301-10 Globalization, coca-colonization and the chronic disease epidemic: can the Doomsday scenario be averted? Zimmet P. International Diabetes Institute, Melbourne, Australia. There are at present approximately 110 million people with diabetes in the world but this number will reach over 220 million by the year 2010, the majority of them with type 2 diabetes. Thus there is an urgent need for strategies to prevent the emerging global epidemic of type 2 diabetes to be implemented. Tackling diabetes must be part of an integrated program that addresses lifestyle related disorders. The prevention and control of type 2 diabetes and the other major noncommunicable diseases (NCDs) can be cost- and health-effective through an integrated (i.e. horizontal) approach to noncommunicable diseases disease prevention and control. With the re-emergence of devastating communicable diseases including AIDS, the Ebola virus and tuberculosis, the pressure is on international and regional agencies to see that the noncommunicable disease epidemic is addressed. The international diabetes and public health communities need to adopt a more pragmatic view of the epidemic of type 2 diabetes and other noncommunicable diseases. The current situation is a symptom of globalization with respect to its social, cultural, economic and political significance.

J Natl Cancer Inst Monogr 1998;(23):23-5 Association of non-acquired immunodeficiency syndrome-defining cancers with human immunodeficiency virus infection. Rabkin CS. Division of Cancer Epidemiology and Genetics, National Cancer Institute, Bethesda, MD, USA. Kaposi's sarcoma and non-Hodgkin's lymphoma were among the earliest recognized manifestations of the acquired immunodeficiency syndrome (AIDS) epidemic. Excluding these two tumors, the overall risk of all other cancers in human immunodeficiency virus (HIV)-infected individuals is similar to that of the general population.

J Natl Med Assoc 1992 Sep;84(9):755-70 AIDS/HIV crisis in developing countries: the need for greater understanding and innovative health promotion approaches. Livingston IL. Department of Sociology/Anthropology, Howard University, Washington, DC 20059. Epidemiologic data on morbidity and mortality have shown that the acquired immunodeficiency syndrome/human immunodeficiency virus (AIDS/HIV) epidemic is relatively widespread in the developing countries of the world, especially in the already economically deprived regions of Sub-Saharan Africa. Africa is estimated to have approximately 5 million seropositive individuals, and by the year

2000, this number is expected to include 10 million HIV-infected children. Improved control over this epidemic can only come through a greater understanding of the specifics of the disease and, eventually, the introduction of more effective and innovative health promotion campaigns targeted at medical personnel, traditional healers, families, and persons with AIDS. Comprehensive health promotion campaigns, carefully using mass media strategies in addition to more community-based programs, all operating under "decentralized" AIDS control programs, are reasoned to be the most efficacious approach that African and other developing countries can use to successfully contain the AIDS/HIV epidemic.

J Nutr 2001 Sep;131(9):2424S-8S Nutrition among older adults in Africa: the situation at the beginning of the millenium. Charlton KE, Rose D. Nutrition & Dietetics Unit, Department of Medicine, University of Cape Town, Cape Town, South Africa. kc@uctgsh1.uct.ac.za Most Africans enter old age after a lifetime of poverty and deprivation, pooraccess to health care and a diet that is usually inadequate in quantity and quality. However, nutrition interventions in African countries are directed primarily toward infants and young children, as well as pregnant and lactating women. This situational analysis focuses on two key areas to identify priorities for future research and policy development: the nutritional status of older Africans and determinants of undernutrition. Based on the scant evidence available, the prevalence of undernutrition is high in older African men (9.5-36.1%) and women (13.1-27%); however, in some urban areas there is evidence that older adults are experiencing the nutrition transition. Information on micronutrient status is sparse, yet it appears that anemia related to suboptimal folate status is a particular problem. Important determinants of poor nutritional status in the elderly in the African context include inadequate household food security, war and famine, and the indirect impact of HIV infection and AIDS.

J R Coll Physicians Lond 1997 Jul-Aug;31(4):425-33 Sun, sex and responsibility. The Lumleian Lecture 1996. Adler MW. Department of Sexually Transmitted Diseases, University College London Medical School.

J Reprod Immunol 1998 Dec;41(1-2):3-15 AIDS and reproductive health. Coggins C, Segal S. The Population Council, New York, NY 10017, USA. ccoggins@popcouncil.org Over 24 million adults worldwide have been infected with HIV. Primarily a sexually transmitted disease, AIDS is inexorably linked to reproductive health and care. Because HIV tends to infect those who are in their reproductive years, the impact of this disease on population growth and life expectancy is projected to be immense in some parts of the world, especially in sub-Saharan Africa. Not least is the challenge to individual families and infant care programs to care for AIDS babies.

JAMA 1992 Sep 23-30;268(12):1581-7 Tuberculosis and HIV infection in sub-Saharan Africa. De Cock KM, Soro B, Coulibaly IM, Lucas SB. Projet RETRO-CI, Abidjan, Ivory Coast. OBJECTIVES--To review the epidemiologic, clinical, and pathological characteristics and the public health implications of human immunodeficiency virus (HIV)-associated tuberculosis in sub-Saharan Africa. DATA CONCLUSIONS--The epidemiology of tuberculosis has been profoundly influenced by the epidemic of HIV infection in sub-Saharan Africa. Greatly increased human and material resources are required for this neglected problem in international health.

Lakartidningen 1996 Jun 5;93(23):2230, 2235-6 Two different HIV types are known. The differences may explain mechanisms of the infection [Article in Swedish] Andersson S, Naucler A, Norrgren H, Biberfeld G. Enheten for immunologi, Smittskyddsinstitutet, Stockholm.

Lancet 1993 Oct 23;342(8878):1037-9 Comment in: Lancet. 1993 Dec 18-25;342(8886-8887):1550. The clinical challenge of the HIV epidemic in the developing world. Gilks CF. Liverpool School of Tropical Medicine, UK.

Lancet 2000 Jun 10;355(9220):2061-6 Accelerating the development and future availability of HIV-1 vaccines: why, when, where, and how? Esparza J, Bhamarapravati N. WHO-UNAIDS HIV Vaccine Initiative, Health Technology and Pharmaceuticals, WHO, Geneva, Switzerland. esparzaj@unaids.org An HIV-1 vaccine offers the best long-term hope to control the AIDS pandemic, especially in less-developed countries. To ensure its future availability we need to increase our research efforts today, including clinical trials. Although small-scale clinical trials of HIV-1 vaccines have been underway since 1987, the first phase III efficacy trials started only recently in the USA and Thailand. Initial results from these trials will be available within the next 2-3 years, and we must start planning now how vaccines should be used if found to be effective. In the meantime, the continuing promotion of the parallel development and assessment of other candidate vaccines is important.

Lancet 2001 May 12;357(9267):1519-23 Comment in: Lancet. 2001 Sep 22;358(9286):1010-1. Deaths from tuberculosis in sub-Saharan African countries with a high prevalence of HIV-1. Harries AD, Hargreaves NJ, Kemp J, Jindani A, Enarson DA, Maher D, Salaniponi FM. National Tuberculosis Control Programme, Ministry of Health, British High Commission, PO Box 30042, Lilongwe 3, Lilongwe, Malawi. adharries@malawi.net

Med Hypotheses 1993 Oct;41(4):289-99 The origin of HIV-1, the AIDS virus. Siefkes D. This article proposes a series of experiments to determine if cows and sheep could be used as animal models for HIV-1, the AIDS virus. To justify this effort, a substantial case is presented that HIV-1 is a natural recombinant of Bovine Leukemia Virus (BLV) and Visna Virus. This natural recombinant may have been inadvertently transferred to humans through the Intensified Smallpox Eradication Program conducted in sub-Saharan Africa in the late 1960s and most of the 1970s.

Med Hypotheses 1997 May;48(5):367-74 The African polio vaccine-acquired immune deficiency syndrome connection. Reinhardt V, Roberts A. Animal Welfare Institute, Washington, DC 20007, USA. Seroepidemiological, clinical and molecular findings suggest that the acquired immune deficiency syndrome virus human immunodeficiency virus-1 was introduced into the human species at the time (late 1950s) and in the geographic ares (Zaire) in which millions of Africans were vaccinated with attenuated poliomyelitis virus strains that were produced in kidney tissue obtained from monkeys. Since monkeys not only harbor viruses that are remarkably similar to and genetically related to human immunodeficiency virus-1, but also served as tissue donors for the African polio vaccine, it is reasonable to suspect that a then non-detectable monkey virus with human-1-like properties was unknowingly co-cultured with the attenuated poliovirus virus and subsequently administered to the vaccinees.

Med J Aust 1996 Nov 4;165(9):494-8 Epidemiology of HIV and AIDS in the Asia-Pacific region. Dore GJ, Kaldor JM, Ungchusak K, Mertens TE. National Centre in HIV Epidemiology and Clinical Research, University of New South Wales, Sydney. The incidence of new HIV infections in Asia and the Pacific will soon pass that in Africa and is projected to increase into the next century. The AIDS epidemic arising from these infections will have enormous consequences for the health and socioeconomic development of a region encompassing more than half the world's population.

Med Law 2000;19(2):287-307 A review of health and human rights after five years of democracy in South Africa. Sarkin J. Law Faculty, University of the Western Cape, South Africa. South Africa became a democratic state with a supreme Constitution and Bill of Rights in 1994. Between 1994 and 1996 South Africans drafted a new constitution which came into force in 1997. While, the right to health, as well as socio-economic rights is provided for, the health care system in post-apartheid South Africa still mirrors that which existed during the apartheid years. There are still two health care systems. The poorly funded public sector services themajority, while the well-funded private sector services the privileged few. A lack of resources is blamed by the state for its inability to provide better and more widespread health services. This article examines, from a human rights perspective, the successes and challenges in developing the right to health between 1994 to 1999, and provides an overview of the present state of health in South Africa.

Med Mycol 2000;38 Suppl 1:259-67

Mycoses in AIDS. Dupont B, Crewe Brown HH, Westermann K, Martins MD, Rex JH, Lortholary O, Kauffmann CA. Unite de Mycologie, Institut Pasteur, H pital Necker, Paris, France. bdupont@pasteur.fr Major changes are occurring in the epidemiology of opportunistic infections (OI) in patients with acquired immune deficiency syndrome (AIDS) and treated with highly active antiretroviral therapy (HAART). A marked decrease of minor and major OI was observed and clinical resistance of thrush to antifungal agents became extremely rare. Primary and secondary prophylaxis against Pneumocystis carinii infections can be stopped; however, the situation is less clear for other OI such as cryptococcosis or endemic mycoses. The epidemiology is dramatically different in the countries which cannot afford the cost of HAART for the majority of patients, such as South Africa. These topics will be discussed in this paper.

Med Mycol 2000;38 Suppl 1:269-79 Mycoses associated with AIDS in the Third World. Marques SA, Robles AM, Tortorano AM, Tuculet MA, Negroni R, Mendes RP. Departamento de Dermatologia, Faculdade de Medicina de Botucatu-UNESP, Brazil. smarques@fmb.unesp.br Despite advances in diagnosis and treatment, the epidemiological status of the human immunodeficiency virus (HIV) infection is far from under control in most of the developing world. Sub-Saharan Africa, Southeast Asia and India show increased rates of new infections.

Med Pregl 1998 Jul-Aug;51(7-8):325-8 Perinatal infection with the human immunodeficiency virus [Article in Serbo-Croatian (Roman)] Milosevic S. Klinika za ginekologiju i akuserstvo, Medicinski fakultet, Novi Sad. INTRODUCTION: HIV infection, eventually resulting in AIDS, represents an important problem of the present days, whereas statistical parameters corresponding with the incidence of its manifestations and lethal outcome deserve great attention and cause anxieity of both general population and medical workers of all profiles. The problem is particularly complicated in the HIV-infected pregnant women. The aim of this paper is to examine epidemiology of HIV and AIDS, influence of HIV infection on the course and outcome of pregnancy, ways of transmission of HIV infection from mother to child, possible effects of progression of HIV infection and medical procedures and approaches in HIV-infected pregnant women. CONCLUSION: HIV infection, reproduction and motherhood jeopardize millions of women worldwide. The most appropriate approach in preventing perinatal transmission involves preventing HIV-1 infection in women of childbearing age, including sexual education nd condom promotion at a very young age.

Med Trop (Mars) 1992 Oct-Dec;52(4):435-8 Cryptococcosis caused by Cryptococcus neoformans var. Gattii. A case associated with acquired immunodeficiency syndrome (AIDS) in Kinshasa, Zaire [Article in French] Muyembe Tamfum JJ, Mupapa Kibadi D, Nganda L, Ngwala-Bikindu D, Kuezina T, Kela-We I, Vandepitte J. Departement de Microbiologie, Universite de Kinshasa, Zaire. Since the introduction of AIDS, the biovar neoformans of Cryptococcus neoformans has replaced the biovar gattii as the predominant agent of cryptococcal meningitis in Kinshasa and in other tropical areas. That this is not an absolute rule is demonstrated by the present case of a HIV-positive patient, observed at the Kinshasa University Hospital, with cryptococcal meningitis due to the biovar gattii. Only four cases of this association have been published before. The authors conclude that both biovars are capable of infecting HIV-positive patients but that the apparent decline of the biovar gattii is related to the rarity of its natural reservoir in the urban environment, where the AIDS epidemic is concentrated.

Med Trop (Mars) 1993 Jan-Mar;53(1):33-43 Ancient serological traces of infections by the human immunodeficiency virus HIV-1 and HIV-2 in sub-saharan Africa. A different geography [Article in French] Remy G. Ecole des Hautes Etudes en Sciences Sociales, Marseille. Despite of some heavy methodological limitations, the analysis of some serological data collected before 1985 allows to establish the selective regional distribution of the two infections. HIV-2 is prevalent in the West African sites which are studied and he has been observed since the sixties. The foci and the sporadic cases of the HIV-1 which are known are localized principally in the East-Central Africa. (Research done under the sponsorship of the A.N.R.S. (Paris)).

Med Trop (Mars) 1993 Jan-Mar;53(1):45-53 The pathogenicity of the human immunodeficiency virus HIV-2 as seen by epidemiologists [Article in French] Soro BN, Gershy-Damet GM, Rey JL. Service d'Epidemiologie-Institut National de Sante Publique, Abidjan-Cote d'Ivoire. The purpose of this study is an evaluation of HIV-2 pathogenicity through an epidemiological analysis, specially in Africa. It is acknowledged that the incubation, or more specially the lapse of time between the infection and the AIDS disease, is longer with HIV-2 than with HIV-1. More over, a certain number of surveys done in Africa show that the average age is higher with HIV-2 than with HIV-1; this is a regular sign of lower pathogenicity. It appears that the sexual transmission of the virus is the same for the HIV-2 and the HIV-1, but it is less effective from mother to baby. Furthermore this type of virus is less prevalent with AIDS patients or AIDS suspects than the HIV-1; and the follow-up of HIV-2 seropositives show that fewer people fall ill than with the HIV-1. A few signs of AIDS standard diagnosis are less frequent among HIV-2 infected patients than among HIV-1 infected patients. Opportunist or associated infections, like tuberculosis or malnutrition, are less often found in HIV-2 patients.

Med Trop (Mars) 1993 Jan-Mar;53(1):61-7 Infection by the human immunodeficiency virus in the Republic of Djibouti: literature review and regional data [Article in French] Rodier G, Couzineau B, Salah S, Bouloumie J, Parra JP, Fox E, Constantine N, Watts D. US Naval Medical Research Unit n. 3, (NAMRU-3) Le Caire Egypte. The first evidence of HIV infection in Djibouti, East Africa, was found in the spring of 1986; the first case of acquired immunodeficiency syndrome (AIDS) was diagnosed in March 1988; and, as of the end of 1991, 104 cases of AIDS had been reported. HIV-1 infection was predominant. Previously published results of four serosurveys carried out in October 87, June 1998, February 1990, and from January 1991 to April 1991 among high risk groups are presented and compared.

Med Trop (Mars) 1994;54(1):67-74 Tuberculosis at the time of AIDS in sub-Saharan Africa. Experience in a central African country: Burundi [Article in French] Aubry P, Kamanfu G, Mlika-Cabanne N, Nikoyagize E, Fagard C, Niyongabo T, Larouze B. Service de Medecine, Centre Hospitalier Universitaire de Kamenge, Faculte de Medecine de Bujumbura, Burundi.

Med Trop (Mars) 1995;55(2):151-3 Disseminated Histoplasma capsulatum histoplasmosis in African AIDS patients (3 cases) [Article in French] Imbert P, Poizot-Martin I, Lacour JP, Marty P, Dhiver C, Martet G. Service de Pathologie Infectieuse et Tropicale, Hopital d'Instruction des Armees LAVERAN, Marseille, France. The authors describe three cases of Histoplasma capsulatum histoplasmosis that occurred in black AIDS patients living in France but originally from Guinea and Ivory Coast. In all three cases histoplasmosis was disseminated with fever. In two cases there were cutaneous manifestations. One patient had renal insufficiency and nephrotic syndrome and another presented ulcerative colitis with histoplasma in the chorion. The outcome was favorable in two patients. These three cases are in addition to the five previously reported cases in african AIDS patients. These cases stress the need for awareness of this opportunistic infection as a complication of AIDS in patients from Black Africa.

Med Trop (Mars) 1998;58(3):297-306 Tropical myositis [Article in French] Saissy JM, Ducourau JP, Tchoua R, Diatta B. Departement d'Anesthesie-Reanimation, l'Hopital d'Instruction des Armees Begin, Saint-Mande, France. Tropical pyomyositis (TP) is a microbial infection involving one or more skeletal muscles that rapidly leads to abscess. The most common infectious agent is Staphylococcus aureus. Since muscle tissue is highly resistant to infection, occurrence of TP is contingent upon one or more compromising factors such as trauma, skin lesions, parasitosis, or malnutrition. HIV infection is currently a major factor in the occurrence of TP.

Med Trop (Mars) 1999;59(2 Suppl):57-9 Present status of HIV infection in Sub-Saharan Africa [Article in French] Delaporte E. Service des Maladies Infectieuses et Tropicales, Centre Hospitalier

Universitaire Gui de Chauliac, Montpellier, France.

Med Trop (Mars) 1999;59(4 Pt 2):449-55 Genetic diversity of HIV infection worldwide and its consequences [Article in French] Peeters M, Delaporte E. Laboratoire des Retrovirus, l'Institut de Recherche pour le Developpement, Montpellier, France. Eric.delaporte@mpl.ird.fr Phylogenetic study of HIV-1 strains from different geographical locations has revealed the existence of three separate groups that have been named M, N, and O. Most strains involved in the pandemia belong to group M which contains several subtypes. Nearly 20 p. 100 of isolates in group M are recombinant with genomic components from different subtypes. Some mosaic virus are one-of-a-kind or limited to small transmission groups while others are major players in the worldwide AIDS epidemic. They are currently called circulating recombinant forms (CRFs). Since subtypes or CRFs must be similar over the whole genome, only 9 subtypes are possible within group M (A, B, C, D, F, G, H, J and K). Viruses E and I in the envelope are recombinant. Subtyping is a powerful molecular tool for monitoring the evolution of the HIV-1 epidemic. Overall the predominant viral forms in the world are subtypes A and C followed by recombinant CRF01-AE (formerly subtype E) and CRF02-AG (identical to the IBNG prototype strain in Nigeria) and subtype B. The highest degree of genetic diversity in HIV-1 is observed in Africa where all subtypes and groups can be observed. The geographic distribution of subtypes is subject to constant change. Recombinant forms of the virus will continue to appear as long as the different subtypes of HIV-1 continue to circulate between continents and recombination continues to occur.

Med Trop (Mars) 1999;59(4 Pt 2):465-7 The HIV/AIDS pandemic: African women at the heart of the control program or the difficulties with regard to gender [Article in French] Moulin B, Louis JP. Mission du Service de Sante des Armees au Ministere des Affaires Etrangeres, Paris, France. bmoulin@hotmail.com The AIDS pandemia in developing countries forces forth the question of women's rights in Africa and underscores their extreme physical and sociocultural vulnerability.

Experience gained during a program designed to reduce mother-to-child transmission of HIV in the Ivory Coast highlights the socially imposed and therefore intricate nature of differences between men and women and of the resulting relationships. Defending a woman's right to know her serologic status empowers her in the fight for emancipation but can also make her more fragile by undermining support from medical staff and family environment.

Med Trop (Mars) 2000;60(4):357-60 Cerebromeningeal listeriosis associated with a cytolytic hepatitis. First case report in Senegal [Article in French] Camara P, Petrognani R, Aubron C, Colbachini P, Ferret C, Hovette P. Service de Medecine Interne et de Pathologies Infectieuses, BP 3006, Hopital Principal, Dakar, Senegal. hovette.p@metissacana.sn Hepatitis due to Listeria monocytogenes is uncommon in adults. This report describes the first case observed in Senegal.

Med Trop (Mars) 2001;61(2):187-93 Co-infections of leishmania/HIV in south Europe [Article in French] Desjeux P, Piot B, O'Neill K, Meert JP.

Departement de Surveillance et Reponse des Maladies transmissibles, Organisation Mondiale de la Sante (OMS), Geneve, Suisse. The Leishmania/HIV co-infection has emerged as a result of the increasing overlap between leishmaniasis (mainly visceral, more rarely cutaneous) and AIDS, which is due to the spread of the AIDS pandemic to rural areas and that of visceral leishmaniasis to suburban areas.

Med Trop (Mars). 1999;59(2):193-200 Leishmaniasis and human immunodeficiency virus: an emerging co-infection? [Article in French] Marlier S, Menard G, Gisserot O, Kologo K, De Jaureguiberry JP. Services Medicaux, l'Hopital d'Instruction des Armees Sainte-Anne, Toulon, France. Although not considered as indicative of AIDS, leishmaniasis presents a number of epidemiologic and clinical features that promote opportunistic infection in HIV patients. Accurate assessment of the incidence of this type of co-infection is difficult due to underestimation in endemic areas such as Africa and Asia. In these areas the WHO estimates that 2 to 9 p. 100 of HIV patients will develop leishmaniasis/HIV co-infection which could become a major concern.

Mol Pathol 2002 Feb;55(1):19-24
Postmodern cancer: the role of human immunodeficiency virus in uterine cervical cancer. Clarke B, Chetty R. Department of Anatomical Pathology, Nelson R Mandela Medical School, School of Pathology and Laboratory Medicine, Congella, 4013, Durban, Natal, South Africa. blaiseclar@hotmail.com The association between cervical cancer and human papillomavirus (HPV) is well known, but its association with human immunodeficiency virus (HIV) is controversial. Coinfection with HPV and HIV is to be expected and recent epidemiological data from Africa show that cervical cancer is the most common AIDS defining neoplasm in women. Unlike other AIDS defining neoplasms, the occurrence of cervical cancer is not dependent on immune compromise. HIV alters the natural history of HPV infection, with decreased regression rates and more rapid progression to high grade and invasive lesions, which are refractory to treatment, requiring more stringent intervention and monitoring.

Mund Kiefer Gesichtschir 1999 Sep;3(5):236-41 Infections of the mouth mucosa (I). HIV infection--an epidemiological, clinical and therapeutic update [Article in German] Reichart PA. Abteilung für Oralchirurgie und zahnarztliche Rontgenologie, Universitatsklinikum Charite, Berlin. peter-a.reichart@charite.de Infections of the oral mucosa have become important with respect to acquired immunodeficiency syndrome (AIDS), particularly as opportunistic infections. In the first part of this overview the epidemiologic, clinical and therapeutical aspects of the HIV infection are addressed. By the end of 1998, WHO had registered 2 million cases of AIDS globally and 33.4 million HIV infections were estimated. Every day 16,000 new infections occur worldwide. Sub-Saharan Africa is the region which has been affected most. By the end of 1998, 18,000 cases of AIDS were registered in Germany, with an estimated 50,000-60,000 HIV infections. The majority of new infections was registered among homosexual men; however, heterosexual transmissions are increasing. Antiretroviral combination therapies had an impact on the clinical course of HIV infection, affecting both mortality and morbidity. The effectiveness of antiretroviral therapy is monitored by determination of the viral load in plasma and CD4(+)-cell counts.

Nature 2001 Apr 19;410(6831):968-73 The global impact of HIV/AIDS. Piot P, Bartos M, Ghys PD, Walker N, Schwartlander B. Joint United Nations Programme on HIV/AIDS (UNAIDS), 20 avenue Appia, 1211 Geneva 27, Switzerland. The scale of the human immunodeficiency virus (HIV)/AIDS epidemic has exceeded all expectations since its identification 20 years ago. Globally, an estimated 36 million people are currently living with HIV, and some 20 million people have already died, with the worst of the epidemic centred on sub-Saharan Africa. But just as the spread of HIV has been greater than predicted, so too has been its impact on social capital, population structure and economic growth. Responding to AIDS on a scale commensurate with the epidemic is a global imperative, and the tools for an effective response are known. Nothing less than a sustained social mobilization is necessary to combat one of the most serious crises facing human

development.

Ned Tijdschr Geneeskd 2000 Dec 2;144(49):2363-7 AIDS: the world's future is in 'their' hands, but comes from 'our' pockets; an impression from the World AIDS Conference in South Africa [Article in Dutch] Veeken H. Artsen zonder Grenzen, Medische afdeling, Postbus 10.014, 1001 EA Amsterdam. hans_veeken@amsterdam.msf.org The HIV-Aids epidemic is a global disaster with vast social, economic, psychological and medical implications. With 34 million persons infected and 19 million cumulative deaths since the start of the epidemic, its impact surpasses all other diseases. The end of the epidemic is not in sight and we will see an increase of HIV cases during the next decennia before the epidemic levels off. This warrants a global solution. Small, nongovernmental projects can never curb this epidemic. The world has to establish a 'global fund', which allocates the resources on a nationwide scale.

Ned Tijdschr Geneeskd 2001 Jun 30;145(26):1236-40 Comment on: Ned Tijdschr Geneeskd. 2001 Jun 30;145(26):1261-5. Results from the 'Ethiopia-

Netherlands AIDS Research Project'; 1995-2000 [Article in Dutch] de Wit TF, Sanders EJ, Fontanet AL, Goudsmit J, Miedema F, Coutinho RA. Ethiopia-Netherlands AIDS Research Project, Ethiopian Health and Nutrition Research Institute, Addis Abeba, Ethiopie. Since 1995 the 'Ethiopia-Netherlands aids research project' (ENARP) has been up and running in Addis Ababa, Ethiopia. Several surveys point towards an HIV seroprevalence of approximately 15% amongst adult Ethiopians in the capital city. Prospective cohort studies initiated since early 1997 indicate that healthy, HIV negative Ethiopians have lower CD4+ T-cell counts compared to the Dutch population and in addition they have chronically activated immune systems, possibly as a result of the highly prevalent intestinal parasitic infections as well as other infections.

Ned Tijdschr Geneeskd 2001 Jun 30;145(26):1261-5 Comment in: Ned Tijdschr Geneeskd. 2001 Jun 30;145(26):1236-40. Ethiopia-Netherlands AIDS research project [Article in Dutch] Sanders EJ, de Wit TF, Fontanet AL, Goudsmit J, Miedema F, Coutinho RA. Ethiopia-Netherlands AIDS

Research Project, Ethiopian Health and Nutrition Research Institute, P.O. Box 1242, Addis Abeba, Ethiopie. eduard@enarp.com The 'Ethiopia-Netherlands AIDS Research Project' (ENARP), started in 1994, is a long-term collaboration between AIDS researchers in Amsterdam and the Ethiopian Health and Nutrition Research Institute in Addis Ababa. The ENARP's primary objectives include conducting studies on HIV and AIDS in Ethiopia, especially by means of some large-scale prospective cohort studies, training Ethiopian scientists in PhD programmes in epidemiology, immunology and virology and establishing a reference laboratory for HIV and AIDS in Ethiopia and neighbouring countries. External funding for ENARP amounts to 32 million Dutch guilders for two periods of four years and is being provided by the Dutch Government. ENARP is the largest third world biomedical project supported by the Dutch Government. In 2000 two Ethiopian students obtained their doctorates from the University of Amsterdam. Five new PhD students commenced their training in 1999. ENARP hopes to set up HIV-1 vaccine phase I and phase II trials in the near future.

Nippon Hoigaku Zasshi 1998 Feb;52(1):51-7 Forensic medicine in Dar-es-Salaam, United Republic of Tanzania [Article in Japanese] Kibayashi K, Tsunenari S. Department of Forensic Medicine, Kumamoto University School of Medicine, Japan. The authors had opportunities to visit and see the present state of forensic medicine in Dar-es-Salaam, a capital city of United Republic of Tanzania. In this city, Department of Histopathology and Morbid Anatomy in Muhimbili University College of Health Sciences is in charge of education and practice of forensic medicine. All bodies of unusual death, about 3,000 cases per year, are brought to the university mortuary and examined by pathologists.

Nurs Clin North Am 1996 Mar;31(1):155-64 Overview of perinatally transmitted HIV infection. Boland M. School of Nursing, University of Medicine and Dentistry of New Jersey, Newark, USA. Over the past 12 years there have been many advances in the recognition, diagnosis, and treatment of pediatric AIDS as well as the unfolding of a pandemic that is a worldwide concern. Whereas in the United States 1100 cases of pediatric HIV and more than 6000 cases of pediatric AIDS have been reported, the greatest devastation by this disease is occurring in Africa and Asia, where heterosexual transmission of HIV is the most common means of infection. This article discusses prevention of pediatric HIV, major diagnostic and treatment advances, understanding perinatal transmission, and approaches to caring for the child with HIV.

Nutrition 1998 Oct;14(10):767-70 Global issues in pediatric nutrition: AIDS. Ball CS. Department of Child Health, King's College Hospital, London, UK. Nutrition is a final common pathway in chronic disease, and weight loss is a major manifestation of acquired immunodeficiency syndrome (AIDS). In sub-Saharan Africa, studies have shown that 25% of children with malnutrition have human immunodeficiency virus (HIV) infection, although patterns of malnutrition are indistinguishable from those who are HIV negative.

Obstet Gynecol Clin North Am 1997 Dec;24(4):705-29 Women and HIV. Epidemiology and global overview. Fowler MG, Melnick SL, Mathieson BJ.

Efficacy Trials Branch, Division of AIDS, National Institute of Allergy and Infectious Diseases, National Institutes of Health, Bethesda, Maryland, USA. The global HIV-1 epidemic in women continues to expand at an alarming rate. More than 11 million women are currently estimated to be HIV-infected, with the majority living in sub-Saharan Africa. The primary risk factor for HIV infection in women is unprotected heterosexual intercourse. Several cofactors may influence a woman's risk for HIV acquisition. These include the presence of other STDs, the prevalence of HIV in the population, engagement in high-risk sexual behaviors at a young age, an increased number of sexual partners, HIV illness severity in an infected partner, host immunogenetic responses, hormonal and other local effects in the female genital tract, and viral characteristics.

Oncologist 1999;4(4):309-17
Cancers in children infected with the human immunodeficiency virus. Mueller BU. Harvard Medical School, Hunnewell Children's Hospital, Boston, Massachusetts 02115, USA. mueller_b@al.tch.harvard.edu The AIDS epidemic continues unabated in Africa, Asia, and South America, and since patients survive longer, the number of chronically immunocompromised individuals is increasing in Europe and the United States. The number of children with HIV infection who will ultimately develop a malignancy is not known. Currently, tumors represent about 2% of the AIDS-defining events in children in the United States, but the incidence might be different in developing countries.

Oral Dis 1997 May;3 Suppl 1:S1-6
The HIV global pandemic: the development and emerging implication. Scully C. Eastman Dental Institute for Oral Health Care Sciences, University of London, UK. AIDS was first observed in 1981. The World Health Organisation has estimated that over 6 million AIDS cases had occurred by late 1995 but that only one-third had been reported. There is an annual increase world-wide of 20%, but in Asia it is in excess of 150% each year. HIV-1 can be classified into two major groups: M which contains 10 subtypes and O which contains several heterogenous viruses. HIV-2, found mainly in Africa, contains at least five subtypes.

Combination therapies with nucleoside analogues are now recommended.

Oral Dis 1997 May;3 Suppl 1:S18-27 Erratum in: Oral Dis 1997 Sep;3(3):206 Epidemiology of HIV-related oral manifestations in women: a review. Shiboski CH. Department of Stomatology, University of California, San Francisco 94143-0422, USA.
OBJECTIVE: (1) To assess the extent of knowledge acquired since 1981 on the epidemiology of HIV-related oral manifestations in women; (2) to determine if these findings differ by gender; and (3) to assess the needs and direction for future epidemiologic research on oral disease and HIV infection in women in relation to men. DATA CONCLUSION: Future epidemiologic studies should be directed at identifying cofactors involved in addition to Epstein-Barr virus (EBV) in the development of hairy leukoplakia, and in addition to KS herpes virus (KSHV) in the occurrence of KS.

P N G Med J 1996 Sep;39(3):190-5 HIV infections in obstetrics and gynaecology. Mola G. Department of Clinical Sciences, Faculty of Medicine, University of Papua New Guinea, Port Moresby, Papua New Guinea.
Thirteen women were discovered to be positive for human immunodeficiency virus (HIV) infection during pregnancy at the Port Moresby General Hospital from 1988 to 1995; of these, eight were diagnosed in the first half of 1995. Risk testing for HIV status is unlikely to discover more than 20% of HIV-positive antenatal patients because risk factors target intravenous drug users and the sexual behaviour of men. Pregnancy does not seem to have a major impact on the progress of HIV disease, but could be detrimental particularly in the later stages of the disease. Especially in developing countries, where HIV-positive patients are more likely to be of poor nutritional status and burdened with a number of other infections, there is a higher risk of preterm labour, small-for-dates babies and chorioamnionitis in pregnancy.

Parasitol Today 1999 Sep;15(9):378-81 Schistosomiasis of the female genital tract: public health aspects. Poggensee G, Feldmeier H, Krantz I. Institut fur Tropenmedizin, Spandauer Damm 130, 14050 Berlin, Germany.

gabriele.poggensee@charite.de In this paper Gabriele Poggensee, Hermann Feldmeier and Ingela Krantz discuss the public health relevance of female genital schistosomiasis (FGS). Some of the stated hypotheses are supported only by clinical observations and/or circumstantial evidence as valid epidemiological and immunological data of this disease entity are still very scanty.

Pathol Biol (Paris) 1994 Nov;42(9):855-60 Free dissociated and precipitated p24 antigenemia of HIV-1 in subjects of the black race [Article in French] Dragon MA, Matta M, Prazuck T, Payan C, Belec L. Laboratoire de Virologie, Hopital Broussais, Paris, France. P24/HIV-1 antigen in the sera from 41 HIV-1-infected Black individuals, living in the Central African Republic (n = 17) and in France (n = 24), and in 21 HIV-1-infected Caucasians patients, matched on the stages of the disease, has been detected and quantified by ELISA, without and with acid pretreatment of the sera by HCl or by glycine, and after ultracentrifugation of serum. Free p24 antigenemia was detected less frequently in Black patients (9.7%), than in Caucasian controls (33%) (p < 0.05). Decomplexed p24 antigenemia was detected in 34% of patients after dissociation of circulating immune complexes (CIC) by HCl (p < 0.01) and in 44% of patients after dissociation of CIC by glycine (p < 0.001). However, the mean concentration of decomplexed p24 antigenemia of positive sera was higher after pretreatment by HCl (88 pg/ml) than by glycine (52 pg/ml), suggesting that a strong acid is more convenient than a weak one to disrupt the CIC in Black individuals. After ultracentrifugation of the serum, the detection of p24 antigen was not significantly increased. Acid dissociation of CIC is a usefull method to increase the sensitivity of detection of circulating p24 antigen in HIV-1-infected Black individuals.

Pediatr Pulmonol Suppl 1997;16:157-9 Childhood tuberculosis and infection with the human immunodeficiency virus. BCG immunization for HIV-seropositive newborns. Bonifachich E. Pulmonology Section, Pediatric Hospital Victor J Vilela, Rosario, Argentina.

Pharmacoeconomics 2001;19(9):937-46 The

economics of HIV vaccines: projecting the impact of HIV vaccination of infants in sub-Saharan Africa. Bos JM, Postma MJ. Groningen University Institute for Drug Exploration/Groningen Research Institute for Pharmacy (GUIDE/GRIP), The Netherlands. J.Bos@farm.rug.nl OBJECTIVES: (i) To project vaccine parameters, economic consequences and market size associated with HIV-1 vaccination of infants in sub-Saharan Africa through the Expanded Program on Immunisation (EPI); and (ii) to assess threshold values for price and effectiveness. CONCLUSION: If technological and financial problems associated with the development of an HIV vaccine can be solved, HIV vaccination in Africa could be both cost effective and potentially profitable.

Pharmacotherapy 1997 Jul-Aug;17(4):670-83 Kaposi's sarcoma: advances in tumor biology and pharmacotherapy. Sung JC, Louie SG, Park SY. Department of Pharmaceutical Economics and Policy, School of Pharmacy, University of Southern California, Los Angeles 90033, USA. Kaposi's sarcoma (KS) is a highly vascularized neoplasm that primarily results in raised, highly vascularized lesions. Before the 1980s, KS was a rare disorder that occurred predominantly in elderly men of Mediterranean or Eastern European Jewish descent. With the advent of the acquired immunodeficiency syndrome (AIDS) epidemic, its occurrence has increased dramatically. It can be classified into four types: classic, African endemic, iatrogenic or drug associated, and AIDS related.

Philos Trans R Soc Lond B Biol Sci 2001 Apr 29;356(1408):517-34 Comment in: Philos Trans R Soc Lond B Biol Sci. 2001 Apr 29;356(1408):595-604. Epidemiology and pathogenesis of Kaposi's sarcoma-associated herpesvirus. Boshoff C, Weiss RA. Department of Oncology and Molecular Pathology, The Wolfson Institute for Biomedical Research, Cruciform Building, University College London, Gower Street, London WC1 6BT, UK. c.boshoff@ucl.ac.uk Kaposi's sarcoma (KS) occurs in Europe and the Mediterranean countries (classic KS) and Africa (endemic KS), immunosuppressed patients (iatrogenic or post-transplant KS) and those with acquired immune deficiency syndrome (AIDS), especially among those who acquired human immunodeficiency virus sexually (AIDS-KS). KS-associated herpesvirus (KSHV or HHV-8) is unusual among herpesviruses in having a restricted geographical distribution. Like KS, which it induces in immunosuppressed or elderly people, the virus is prevalent in Africa, in Mediterranean countries, among Jews and Arabs and certain Amerindians. Distinct KSHV genotypes occur in different parts of the world, but have not been identified as having a differential pathogenesis.

Philos Trans R Soc Lond B Biol Sci 2001 Jun 29;356(1410):795-8 Epidemiology and the emergence of human immunodeficiency virus and acquired immune deficiency syndrome. De Cock KM. Centers for Disease Control and Prevention, Kenya, PO Box 30137, Nairobi, Kenya. kdecock@kisian.mimcom.net Although acquired immune deficiency syndrome (AIDS) was first described in the USA in 1981, there is evidence that individual cases occurred considerably earlier in Central Africa, and serological and virological data show human

immunodeficiency virus (HIV) was present in the Democratic Republic of Congo (DRC) as far back as 1959. It is likely that HIV-1 infection in humans was established from cross-species transmission of simian immunodeficiency virus of chimpanzees, but the circumstances surrounding this zoonotic transfer are uncertain. This presentation will review how causality is established in epidemiology, and review the evidence (a putative ecological association) surrounding the hypothesis that early HIV-1 infections were associated with trials of oral polio vaccine (OPV) in the DRC.

Philos Trans R Soc Lond B Biol Sci 2001 Jun 29;356(1410):803-14 Comment in: Philos Trans R Soc Lond B Biol Sci. 2001 Jun 29;356(1410):825-9. Experimental oral polio vaccines and acquired immune deficiency syndrome. Hooper E. Penguin Books, 27 Wrights Lane, London W8 5TZ, UK. The simian immunodeficiency virus (SIV) of the common chimpanzee is widely acknowledged as the direct ancestor of HIV-1. There is increasing historical evidence that during the late 1950s, kidneys were routinely excised from central African chimpanzees by scientists who were collaborating with the polio vaccine research of Dr Hilary Koprowski, and sent - inter alia - to vaccine-making laboratories in the USA and Africa, and to unspecified destinations in Belgium. While there is no direct evidence that cells from these kidneys were used as a substrate for growing Dr Koprowski's oral polio vaccines, there is a startling coincidence between places in Africa where his CHAT vaccine was fed, and the first appearances in the world of HIV-1 group M and group-M-related AIDS.

Philos Trans R Soc Lond B Biol Sci 2001 Jun 29;356(1410):855-66 Using human immunodeficiency virus type 1 sequences to infer historical features of the acquired immune deficiency syndrome epidemic and human immunodeficiency virus evolution. Yusim K, Peeters M, Pybus OG, Bhattacharya T, Delaporte E, Mulanga C, Muldoon M, Theiler J, Korber B. Los Alamos National Laboratory, Los Alamos, PO Box 1663, NM 87545, USA. In earlier work, human immunodeficiency virus type 1 (HIV-1) sequences were analysed to estimate the timing of the ancestral sequence of the main group of HIV-1, the virus that is responsible for the acquired immune deficiency syndrome pandemic, yielding a best estimate of 1931 (95% confidence interval of 1915-1941). That work will be briefly reviewed, outlining how phylogenetic tools were extended to incorporate improved evolutionary models, how the molecular clock model was adapted to incorporate variable periods of latency, and how the approach was validated by correctly estimating the timing of two historically documented dates.

Philos Trans R Soc Lond B Biol Sci 2001 Jun 29;356(1410):923-5 The earliest cases of human immunodeficiency virus type 1 group M in Congo-Kinshasa, Rwanda and Burundi and the origin of acquired immune deficiency syndrome. Vangroenweghe D. The early cases of acquired immune deficiency syndrome and human immunodeficiency virus type 1 (HIV-1) infection in the 1960s and 1970s in Congo-Kinshasa (Zaire), Rwanda and Burundi are reviewed. These countries appear to be the source of the HIV-1 group M epidemic, which then spread outwards to neighbouring Tanzania and Uganda in the east, and Congo-

Brazzaville in the west. Further spread to Haiti and onwards to the USA can be explained by the hundreds of single men from Haiti who participated in the UNESCO educational programme in the Congo between 1960 and 1975.

Philos Trans R Soc Lond B Biol Sci 2001 Jun 29;356(1410):939-43 The burden of proof and the origin of acquired immune deficiency syndrome. Martin B. Science, Technology and Society, University of Wollongong, New South Wales 2522, Australia. brian_martin@uow.edu.au There is a distinct difference in the way that different theories about the origin of acquired immune deficiency syndrome have been treated, with the widely supported cut-hunter theory given relatively little scrutiny, while the oral polio vaccine theory has been subject to intense criticism. This difference in treatment cannot be explained as application of the scientific method. A better explanation is that the burden of proof is put on all contenders to the cut-hunter theory, giving it an unfair advantage, especially given that this assignment of the burden of proof appears to reflect non-scientific factors.

Practitioner 1997 Jan;241(1570):16, 20-2, 25-6 Tuberculosis: the case for vigilance. Ormerod P.

Presse Med 1992 Sep 26;21(31):1476-81 Infectious respiratory complications of AIDS [Article in French] Bouvet E. Clinique de Reanimation des Maladies infectieuses, Hopital Bichat-Claude Bernard, Paris. Respiratory infections are particularly frequent in HIV infection. They depend upon the degree of immunodeficiency, the geographical region and a possible prophylaxis. Bronchopneumopathies caused by pyogenic organisms (notably pneumococci) appear when the number of T4 lymphocytes is little reduced. Pulmonary tuberculosis, particularly frequent in Africans and Haitians, occurs in patients with moderate immunodeficiency (T4 between 200 and 300/mm3). HIV infections modify the epidemiology of tuberculosis in Africa, but also in the USA and probably in Europe.

Presse Med 2000 Jan 29;29(3):146-52 HIV infection in Africa. Clinical and therapeutical research [Article in French] Salamon R, Anglaret X, Leroy V, Dabis F. Unite INSERM 330, Universite Victor Segalen

Bordeaux 2.
Roger.Salamon@dim.u-
bordeaux2.fr A MAJOR
HEALTH PROBLEM: Human
Immunodeficiency Virus (HIV)
infection is a major public
health problem in sub-Saharan
Africa and the care of HIV-
infected patients is limited by
the lack of resources. Clinical
research can play a major role to
assess the benefit of preventive
and/or curative measures
adapted to the context of these
countries. To illustrate advances
and gaps in HIV/AIDS clinical
research in Africa, we explored
three issues relevant to this
research: opportunistic
infections in adults, mother-to-
child transmission of HIV and
the ethical questions.
PREVENTION: Prevention of
mother-to-child transmission
and care of HIV+ adults in the
area of opportunistic infections
are feasible in Africa with an
acceptable cost. This requires
first to train and inform health
care providers and the
populations. Lots of
uncertainties in these areas are
likely to be alleviated by
reinforcing clinical and
therapeutic research of good
quality including the questions
of antiretroviral treatment.
Ethical issues raised by the
design and conduct of clinical
research in Africa need a

positive thinking to face the
HIV African pandemic.

Psychiatry Clin Neurosci 1995
May;49 Suppl 1:S117-21
Psychopathology and
psychotherapy in the dying
AIDS patient. O'Dowd MA.
Albert Einstein College of
Medicine, Montefiore Medical
Center, New York 10467, USA.
Although this paper deals with
the dying AIDS patient, some of
the issues faced by the therapist
working with any population of
dying patients will be reviewed
before focusing more
specifically, on some of the
particular issues seen in working
with AIDS patients.

Q J Nucl Med 1995 Sep;39(3):169-
86 Role of nuclear medicine
and AIDS: overview and
perspective for the future. Ganz
WI, Serafini AN. Department of
Radiology, University of Miami
School of Medicine, Florida
33101, USA. The Human
Immunodeficiency Virus (HIV)
is the causative agent for the
expanding epidemic of the
Acquired Immunodeficiency
Syndrome (AIDS). Sixteen
million individuals were
estimated to be infected
worldwide with HIV by the
World Health Organization in
1995, with over 10 million in
Africa and one million in the

USA. As the HIV cost in dollars and lives continues to rise it will become more important to understand AIDS and to foresee the potential role of nuclear medicine in HIV diseases. Nuclear medicine may have a role in the assessment of immune function, including the ability to predict if individuals can avoid progression to HIV+status, if pre-AIDS to AIDS conversion can be prevented, and if an individual's immune status requires addition of prophylaxis. Also it can be used for disease detection at an early stage and determination of the extent of disease. It is especially useful to assist clinicians in optimizing therapy and assessing its efficacy. In the future new radiopharmaceuticals for detecting a specific infections and tumors will be needed.

Reprod Health Matters 2001 Nov;9(18):143-55 Male circumcision as an HIV control strategy: not a 'natural condom'. Bonner K. Graduate Entry Programme, St George's Hospital Medical School, Cranmer Terrace, London SW17 0RE, UK. pg004596@sghms.ac.uk Recent epidemiological studies have shown fairly convincingly that in high-risk populations in sub-Saharan Africa, male circumcision is associated with a reduced risk of HIV infection. Following a consultation at the XIII International AIDS Conference in July 2000 in Durban, there was growing interest in such an intervention. This paper explores what is known about male circumcision, the risks associated with it, its relationship with sexual health, including HIV and other sexually transmitted infections (STIs), and the potential problems with implementing circumcision as an intervention internationally, particularly in traditionally non-circumcising communities and those where access to medical facilities is limited.

Respirology 1997 Sep;2(3):209-13 Tuberculosis and HIV infection: global perspectives. Murray JF. Division of Pulmonary and Critical Care Medicine, San Francisco General Hospital Medical Center, University of California, USA. This paper reviews the epidemiological and clinical aspects of the interaction between Mycobacterium tuberculosis and HIV infection. The incidence of HIV-associated tuberculosis is increasing worldwide and is expected to increase further, especially in Africa and parts of

Asia. HIV infection appears to increase the likelihood that tuberculous infection will occur after tubercle bacilli are inhaled into the lungs. Moreover, there is persuasive evidence that in the presence of HIV infection, new-onset tuberculous infection will progress rapidly to clinically significant disease and the probability that latent tuberculous infection will reactivate is enormously increased. The accelerating and amplifying influence of HIV infection is also contributing to the increasing incidence of disease caused by multidrug-resistant strains of M. tuberculosis. Neither clinical nor radiographic features reliably distinguish the majority of patients with HIV-associated tuberculosis from those who are non-HIV-infected. Some HIV-infected patients, however, have atypical manifestations and are difficult to diagnose.

Rev Clin Esp 1996 Jul;196(7):479-87 Management of viral hepatitis in patients with HIV infection [Article in Spanish] Soriano V, Garcia-Samaniego J. Centro de Investigaciones Clinicas, Instituto de Salud Carlos III, Madrid.

Rev Med Brux 2000 Apr;21(2):75-83 Tuberculosis associated with the human immunodeficiency virus [Article in French] Gerard M. Clinique des Maladies infectieuses, C.H.U. Saint Pierre, U.L.B. The HIV pandemic is one of the factors that have contributed to the the worldwide increase in tuberculosis cases especially in subsaharian Africa. The copathogenicity between M. tuberculosis and HIV is best illustrated by the high susceptibility of the HIV-infected persons for reactivation of a remote tuberculous infection or early progression of a newly acquired disease and by the negative impact of tuberculosis on natural history of HIV characterised by increased incidence of clinical progression and increased mortality rates. Clinical presentation is rather atypical and severe when immune suppression is advanced: no cavitation on the chest X-rays, visceral ganglionnar involvement with frequent fistulization, positive blood cultures.

Rev Med Interne 1993;14(7):715-22 Tuberculosis and HIV [Article in French] Rogeaux O, Bricaire F, Gentilini M. Departement des maladies infectieuses, parasitaires, tropicales et de sante publique CHU Pitie-

Salpetriere, Paris, France. With the increased number of HIV infected patients, tuberculosis has become more frequent in Europe, USA and particularly in Africa. Impaired immunity, poor life conditions and high prevalence of tuberculosis in the general population facilitate the transmission of the disease. Tuberculosis is often seen early in the course of HIV infection and sometimes reveals the underlying immunodeficiency. Most of these cases are due to reactivation of earlier primo-infection when tuberculosis occurs later in the HIV disease, it may be secondary to a recent contagion.

Rev Pneumol Clin 1994;50(5):260-7 Multiresistant tuberculosis [Article in French] Murray JF. Pulmonary and Critical Care Division, San Francisco General Hospital Medical Center, University of California San Francisco. Multiresistant tuberculosis has been recognized since the advent of triple-drug therapy with isoniazid, streptomycin and PAS in the fifties, but the recently observed strains of Mycobacterium tuberculosis resistant both to isoniazid and to rifampicin, the rapid spread of the infection and the development of severe disease

in HIV infected patients have raised grave problems in controlling tuberculosis in the world. The disease is difficult and expansive to treat in industrialized countries and is incurable in many developing countries. The increased prevalence of resistant strains in southeast Asia or in Subsahars Africa is a real disaster as both the incidence of tuberculosis and of HIV infection is high. It is extremely difficult or even impossible to deal with such a disaster without new antituberculosis drugs and improved means of prevention.

Rev Pneumol Clin 1995;51(6):321-4 Standard radiological characteristics of thoracic sites of tuberculosis in patients with AIDS in a Tunisian population [Article in French] Tiouiri H, Louzir B, Ben Salem N, Beji M, Kilani B, Gastli M, Daghfous J, Zribi A. Services des Maladies Infectieuses, CHU La Rabta, Tunis, Tunisie. Aspects of tuberculosis on the standard chest X-ray in a population of 18 AIDS patients in Tunisia were examined. The diagnosis of pulmonary tuberculosis was confirmed in all cases with bacteriology tests. Diffuse lesions of the parenchyma predominated contrasting with the exceptional nature of cavernous formations. Localized infiltrations were infrequent and intrathoracic node enlagement was rare. Cases with no abnormal radiological signs were also seen in advanced HIV infection. Such atypical cases, in agreement with data in the literature, would be explained by immunoradiologic correlation. Thus it is necessary to search for the tuberculosis bacilli in all patients with HIV infection whatever the aspect on the standard chest X-ray.

Rev Pneumol Clin 1997;53(2):79-84 Pulmonary complications of human immunodeficiency virus infection in sub-Saharan Africa [Article in French] Domoua K, N'Dhatz M, Coulibaly G, Traore F, Koffi J, Achi V, Cisse L, Kouame S, Beugre LK, Konan JB, Yapi A. Service de Pneumo-phtisiologie, CHU de Treichville, Abidjan, Cote d'Ivoire. Based on a selection of articles published in the literature and reports from international AIDS conferences, we present the main pulmonary complications of HIV-infection observed in sub-Saharan Africa.

Rev Pneumol Clin 1998 Dec;54(6):311-20 American pulmonary histoplasmosis caused by Histoplasma capsulatum [Article in French] Guigay J, Cuguilliere A, Miltgen J, Lonjon T, Jancovici R, Vaylet F, Natali E, Le Vagueresse R, Bonnet D, L'Her P. Service de Pneumologie, Hopital d'Instruction des Armees Percy, Clamart. American pulmonary histoplasmosis is a deep mycosis imported from North America caused by the inhalation of Histoplasma capsulatum. It is endemic in several countries throughout the world and occasional cases have been reported in France, mainly imported from out lying French territories. The most frequent clinical forms observed in immunocompetent subjects are generally benign or silent and usually limited to a fortuitously discovered pulmonary nodule. Massive exposure may lead to an acute primary invasion producing a miliary aspect. Chronic forms simulating tuberculosis are exceptional. Inversely, opportunistic histoplasmosis in AIDS patients can produce an severe multiple organ disease.

Rev Rhum Ed Fr 1994 Dec;61(11):829-38 Bone and joint sites of African histoplasmosis (Histoplasma duboisii). Apropos of a case and review of the literature [Article in French] Simon F, Chouc PY,

Herve V, Branquet D, Jeandel P. Service de Medecine, Hopital Regional de Bambari, Republique Centrafricaine (1), Marseille Armees. The authors report a case of disseminated African histoplasmosis with bone and joint involvement in a black 28-year-old citizen of the Central African Republic who presented with a 17-month history of multiple osteoarticular lesions (sternoclavicular joints, humerus, ribs), cutaneous lesions (face, scalp, thorax), and lymphadenopathy. Clinical manifestations resolved rapidly under treatment with ketoconazole (600 mg/d for 10 days then 400 mg/day for nine months). Persistent yeast cells were then found upon examination of a lymph node biopsy specimen. The characteristics and diagnosis of osteoarticular lesions due to African histoplasmosis are discussed on the basis of a review of the literature. Bone and joint lesions due to African histoplasmosis have not yet been reported in patients with the acquired immunodeficiency syndrome.

S Afr Med J 1993 Sep;83(9):668-74 AIDS prevention in South Africa. A perspective from other African countries. Wilson D, Lavelle S. Psychology

Department, University of Zimbabwe, Harare.

S Afr Med J 1994 Aug;84(8 Pt 1):503-5 HIV-2 and its neurological manifestations. Rolfe M. Royal Victoria Hospital, Banjul, The Gambia, West Africa. The human immunodeficiency virus type 2 (HIV-2) produces a similar spectrum of illness as HIV-1, including AIDS, and is clinically indistinguishable. There is evidence that it is less pathogenic, with a longer natural history. HIV-2 infection is endemic in West Africa, especially in the former Portuguese and French colonies. Trade, migration, war and tourism have been important factors in the spread of the virus through the subregion and beyond. Diagnostic facilities necessary for the accurate diagnosis of neurological disease are not available in most of Africa and autopsy reports have been few. These constraints have restricted the information available on the pattern of neuropathology induced by HIV-2.

S Afr Med J 1996 Jan;86(1):27-8 HIV/AIDS in South Africa--a relentless progression? McIntyre J.

S Afr Med J 1996 Jan;86(1):55-60
Academic research and
HIV/AIDS in South Africa.
Campbell CM, Williams BG.
London School of Economics
and Political Science, UK.

S Afr Med J 1997 Mar;87(3):285-90
Comment in: S Afr Med J. 1997
Aug;87(8):1015-6. Should
South Africa be preparing for
HIV-1 vaccine efficacy trials?
Morris L, van der Ryst E, Gray
C, Williamson C.

S Afr Med J 2000 Aug;90(8):769-
72 HIV vaccine trials in South
Africa--some ethical
considerations. Lindegger G,
Slack C, Vardas E. Department
of Psychology, University of
Natal, Pietermaritzburg.

S Afr Med J 2001 May;91(5):384-7
Access to essential medications
for HIV/AIDS in South Africa.
Andrews S. Brooklyn Medical
Centre, 379 Koeberg Road,
Rugby, Cape Town.

S Afr Med J 2001 Nov;91(11):948-
51 Progress towards developing
a vaccine to prevent HIV and
AIDs in South Africa. Morris L,
Williamson C, Vardas E. AIDS
Virus Research Unit, National
Institute for Virology,
Johannesburg.

Sante 1996 Nov-Dec;6(6):371-6

Epidemiological portrait of
acquired immunodeficiency
syndrome and its implications in
Benin [Article in French] Fourn
L, Ducic S. Universite nationale
du Benin, Faculte des Sciences
de la Sante, Unite
d'enseignement et de recherche
en sante publique, Cotonou.
This paper describes the
epidemiological pattern of AIDS
and its social, demographic and
economical implications as they
affect the current national
program to increase the
awareness of the problem.

Sante 1997 Mar-Apr;7(2):89-94
Primary chemoprevention of
tuberculosis in HIV-infected
patients in non-industrialized
countries [Article in French]
Anglaret X, Dabis F,
Batungwanayo J, Perronne C,
Taelman H, Bonard D, Sylla-
Koko F, Leroy V, Van de Perre
P, Vilde JL, Salamon R. Centre
de diagnostic et de recherches
surle sida et les infections
opportunistes (CEDRES), CHU
de Treichville, Abidjan, Cote
d'Ivoire. In randomized placebo-
controlled trials in Haiti, Zambia
and Uganda, prophylactic use of
isoniazid (INH) for 6 to 12
months reduced the annual
incidence of tuberculosis in
HIV-infected patients by more
than 50 per cent. For several
years, WHO, IUTATLD and

CDC have recommended that HIV-positive patients testing positive in a PPD test should be treated with INH as a form of anti-tuberculosis chemoprophylaxis (ATC).

Sante 1997 May-Jun;7(3):177-86 How to manage HIV seropositive or AIDS patients in rural Burkina Faso? [Article in French] Taverne B. ORSTOM, Burkina Faso. This article is based on an ethnographical study carried out in 1996. It describes and analyzes the methods of medical and family management of HIV-positive and full-blown AIDS patients in the rural environment of Burkinabe. A number of recommendations are made.

Sante 2001 Jan-Feb;11(1):43-8 Approach to sexuality in an AIDS context in Congo [Article in French] Courtois R, Mullet E, Malvy D. Service de psychiatrie de l'enfant et de l'adolescent, Chateau du Clos Saint-Victor, 3 rue de Chantepie, 37300 Joue-les-Tours, France. The pandemic due to the human immunodeficiency virus (HIV) is extensive in Sub-Saharan Africa and especially in Congo. Congo is a small country on the Atlantic coast and characterized by plentiful equatorial forests and low population density (essentially urban). In Congo, there is a high prevalence of HIV. The social and economic consequences of AIDS add to those of a recent civil war in 1997. There were fratricidal confrontations before and after this period.

Sante Publique 1999 Jun;11(2):155-65 Pregnancy and delivery in western Africa. High risk motherhood [Article in French] Prual A. Ministere de la Sante et des Affaires Sociales, Nouakchott, Republique Islamique de Mauritanie. According to the World Health Organization, 585,000 women die each year from a pregnancy-related cause, 99% of whom are from developing countries. The first International Conference on Safe Motherhood in 1987 sensitized the world community to this drama. Ever since, maternal mortality and its medical causes are better known. The maternal mortality ratio is highest in West Africa (1,020 maternal deaths per 100,000 live borns) when it is 27/100,000 in industrialized countries. Direct obstetric causes account for 80% of the deaths: hemorrhage, infection, dystocia, hypertension and abortion. Indirect causes are essentially anemia, malaria, hepatitis C and AIDS. Severe maternal morbidity is 6 to 10 times more frequent than maternal mortality but it also leads to handicaps which end up often in women's social rejection.

Scand J Gastroenterol Suppl 1996;220:147-52 AIDS in Africa. O'Keefe EA, Wood R. Dept. of Medicine, University of Cape Town, Somerset Hospital, Greenpoint, South Africa. HIV has infected more than 10 million people in sub-Saharan Africa with prevalence rates of up to 30% reported from some countries. Adult transmission of HIV in Africa is mainly heterosexual and over half of new infections are in women. About 40% of infants born to HIV-positive mothers are themselves infected. Diarrhoea occurs in 90% of African AIDS patients and 'slim disease' (prolonged diarrhoea and wasting usually due to coccidian parasites) is pathognomic of AIDS in Central Africa.

Scand J Infect Dis 2001;33(8):563-7 Tuberculosis: trends and the twenty-first century. Arnadottir T. International Union Against Tuberculosis and Lung Disease, Paris, France. The global burden of tuberculosis is enormous, even if estimates are somewhat uncertain. The forces

counteracting control measures, namely demographic factors, drug resistance, HIV, migration, poverty and marginalization, are enormous as well. With accelerated reforms in tuberculosis programs important progress can be made towards the control of tuberculosis early in the 21st century. This is confirmed by studying reports from countries where control measures have been implemented and sustained.

Schweiz Med Wochenschr 1993 Feb 6;123(5):140-7 Tuberculosis 1992: current clinical aspects, epidemiology and diagnosis [Article in German] Rochat T. Division de pneumologie, Hopital cantonal universitaire, Geneve. We review four different aspects of tuberculosis (TB), a disease which is making a comeback as a focus of medical attention. The diagnosis of TB in HIV infected individuals can be very challenging for the clinician and an increased number of side effects complicates treatment. Updated information in this area appears necessary for physicians who are in charge of HIV-infected patients. The "cursed duet" of TB and HIV infection is also responsible for the increase of TB in subsaharan Africa. Recent data are discussed in relation to this issue.

Schweiz Med Wochenschr 1997 Jul 22;127(29-30):1223-8 HIV-associated tuberculosis in Africa exemplified by Zimbabwe [Article in German] Schoch OD. Kliniken A und B fur Innere Medizin, Kantonsspital St. Gallen. In Africa, a rapid increase of human immunodeficiency virus (HIV)-associated tuberculosis cases has been observed; 80% of a worldwide 6 million dually infected persons live in this part of the world. The annual risk of progression to clinically overt tuberculosis in dually infected persons approaches the lifetime risk in persons with tuberculosis but no HIV infection.

Sci Am 2000 Nov;283(5):98-103 AIDS drugs for Africa. Ezzell C.

Sci Total Environ 1996 Nov 22;191(3):245-69 The HIV/AIDS epidemic: its evolutionary implications for human ecology with special reference to the immune system. Caldararo N. Department of Anthropology, San Francisco State University, CA 94132, USA. The epidemiology of AIDS in Africa is discussed. Serological and clinical dats on virology and population genetics are related to current theories of heterosexual transmission and to cultural practices involving the exchange or transmission of body fluids between individuals, such as female and male genital mutilation and indigenous or 'folk' medicine, as well as non-Western medical uses of medical syringes. A review of the relationship of autoimmune conditions, graft-vs-host disease and the retrovirus/oncogene involvement is presented.

Science 2000 Jan 28;287(5453):607-14 AIDS as a zoonosis: scientific and public health implications. Hahn BH, Shaw GM, De Cock KM, Sharp PM. Department of Medicine, Howard Hughes Medical Institute, University of Alabama at Birmingham, Birmingham, AL 35294, USA. bhahn@uab.edu Evidence of simian immunodeficiency virus (SIV) infection has been reported for 26 different species of African nonhuman primates. Two of these viruses, SIVcpz from chimpanzees and SIVsm from sooty mangabeys, are the cause of acquired immunodeficiency syndrome (AIDS) in humans. Together, they have been transmitted to humans on at least seven occasions. The implications of human infection by a diverse set of SIVs and of exposure to a plethora of additional human immunodeficiency virus-related viruses are discussed.

Scott Med J 2000 Oct;45(5 Suppl):47-50; discussion 51 Issues facing TB control (6). Tuberculosis control in sub-Saharan Africa in the face of HIV and AIDS. Harries AD.

Semin Cancer Biol 1999 Jun;9(3):175-85 Seroepidemiology of Kaposi's sarcoma-associated herpesvirus (KSHV). Chatlynne LG, Ablashi DV. Advanced Biotechnologies Inc, Columbia, Maryland 21046, USA. Since the Kaposi's sarcoma-associated herpesvirus (KSHV also referred to as HHV-8, human herpesvirus-8) was discovered it has been shown that the virus is associated with all cases of Kaposi's sarcoma (KS) classical, endemic, or AIDS associated. In the numerous countries where the seroprevalence of this virus has been studied, data demonstrate that the virus is not ubiquitous in general healthy human populations as is the case with other human herpesviruses. Many seroprevalence studies to detect antibodies to HHV-8 have now been conducted using a variety of immunologic techniques. While these assays are not in total agreement and may overstate or understate the positivity of sera in the general population, they all show similar general antibody trends.

Semin Neonatol 2000 Aug;5(3):181-8 HIV in pregnancy: strategies for management. Coovadia HM, Coutsoudis A. Department of Paediatrics and Child Health, University of Natal, Congella, 4013, South Africa. mackrory@med.und.ac.za HIV/AIDS is now the leading cause of mortality in Africa. Measures for preventing HIV infection in women are central to any strategy to manage this disease in pregnancy. The use of anti-retrovirals (ARVs) has reduced vertical transmission in industrialized countries by about two-thirds. Recent ARV trials in developing countries reveal relative efficacies at 6 months of about 40% in breast feeding and 50% in non-breast feeding populations. New data on breast feeding adds to the information on the pathogenesis of postnatal transmission and can influence feeding recommendations. Strategies suitable and inappropriate for developing countries, and operational difficulties, are discussed. Copyright 2000 Harcourt

Publishers Ltd.

Semin Neonatol 2000 Aug;5(3):189-96 Current issues in maternal and perinatal tuberculosis: impact of the HIV-1 epidemic. Thillagavathie P. Department of Paediatrics and Child Health, Medical School, University of Natal, Congella, Durban, 4013, South Africa. pillayti@med.und.ac.za Human immunodeficiency virus type 1 (HIV-1) and tuberculosis (TB) are among the leading causes of disability and death in the developing world, the largest burden borne by sub-Saharan Africa and Asia. Both diseases are significant among women of childbearing age, and TB, although uncommon in pregnancy, is on the increase. While earlier reports were contradictory regarding the effect of TB on the course of pregnancy and vice versa, the negative impacts of each on the other have been documented, some in relation to HIV-1 co-infection. This review focuses on emerging data on maternal and perinatal TB within the context of HIV-1 infection. Copyright 2000 Harcourt Publishers Ltd.

Semin Oncol 2001 Apr;28(2):179-87 Hepatocellular carcinoma in the developing world. Ogunbiyi JO. Department of Pathology, University College Hospital, Ibadan, Nigeria. ogunbiyi@skannet.com There has recently been an observable increase in some forms of cancer the world over. This is attributable in large part to the introduction of acquired immunodeficiency syndrome (AIDS)-related malignancies into the world of medicine and it is interesting that most of these cases are seen in the developing world, which proportionately leads with the number of AIDS cases. Despite this, some more traditional cancers remain the big killers in these areas of the world, except that in some countries definitive interventions have yielded excellent results in reducing disease burden.

Semin Oncol 2001 Apr;28(2):198-206 Acquired immunodeficiency syndrome-associated cancers in Sub-Saharan Africa. Thomas JO. Department of Pathology, University College Hospital, Ibadan, Nigeria. ibadan.canreg@skannet.com Sub-Saharan Africa is considered home to more than 60% of all human immunodeficiency virus (HIV) infected cases, with an estimated adult prevalence of 8.0%. It is stated that this region has contributed more than 90% of childhood deaths related to HIV infection and about 93% of childhood acquired immunodeficiency syndrome (AIDS)-related deaths. Although no country in Africa is spared of the infection, the bulk is seen in East and South Africa, with the highest recorded rates of 20% to 50% in Zimbabwe. On the other hand, West Africa is less affected, while countries in Central Africa have relatively stable infection rates.

Semin Respir Infect 1999 Dec;14(4):327-32 Bacterial pneumonia. Schneider RF. Division of Pulmonary and Critical Care Medicine, Beth Israel Medical Center, Albert Einstein College of Medicine, New York, New York 10003, USA. Bacterial pneumonia is significantly more common in persons who are HIV-infected than in the general population and is most common among injection drug users and in persons with advanced HIV disease and immunosuppression. The clinical features of bacterial pneumonia are similar to those in HIV-seronegative persons, but bacteremia is more common. When a pathogen is identified, Streptococcus pneumoniae is consistently the most common,

occurring in 20% to 70% of cases. Haemophilus influenzae, Staphylococcus aureus, Escherichia coli, and other gram-negative organisms are mainly responsible for the remainder of bacterial pneumonia episodes in the United States, Central Africa, Australia, and England.

Semin Respir Infect 1999 Dec;14(4):366-71 Intensive care of patients with HIV infection. Rosen MJ. Division of Pulmonary and Critical Care Medicine, Beth Israel Medical Center, Albert Einstein College of Medicine, New York, New York 10003, USA. Despite the improvements in the prognosis associated with the development of highly active antiretroviral therapy (HAART), more than 410,000 people in the United States were reported to have died from acquired immune deficiency syndrome (AIDS) by the end of 1998. The number of people living with human immunodeficiency virus (HIV) infection and AIDS in the United States continues to increase, estimated at more than 370,000 in 1998, and there is good reason for optimism that HIV infection may be a controllable disease in many people. Nevertheless, an estimated 27,000 persons still died of AIDS in the United States in 1997, and AIDS is still a leading cause of death in the age group 25 to 44 years. Despite the dramatic treatment advances for HIV infection and improving survival following an AIDS diagnosis, many patients still present with life-threatening complications of HIV infection for three major reasons. Highly active antiretroviral therapy and prophylaxis against Pneumocystis carinii and other infections are not effective in all patients, despite rigorous adherence to treatment. Others adhere to these therapies poorly.

Sex Transm Infect 1999 Feb;75(1):3-17 From epidemiological synergy to public health policy and practice: the contribution of other sexually transmitted diseases to sexual transmission of HIV infection. Fleming DT, Wasserheit JN. Division of STD Prevention, National Center for HIV, STD, and TB Prevention, Centers for Disease Control and Prevention, Atlanta, GA 30333, USA. OBJECTIVES: To review the scientific data on the role of sexually transmitted diseases (STDs) in sexual transmission of HIV infection and discuss the implications of these findings for HIV and STD prevention policy and practice.

METHODS: Articles were selected from a review of Medline, accessed with the OVID search engine. The search covered articles from January 1987 to September 1998 and yielded 2101 articles. Methods used to uncover articles which might have been missed included searching for related articles by author, and combing literature reviews. In addition, all abstracts under the category "sexually transmitted diseases" from the XI and XII International Conferences on AIDS (Vancouver 1996 and Geneva 1998) and other relevant scientific meetings were reviewed. Efforts were made to locate journal articles which resulted from the research reported in the identified abstracts.

Soc Sci Med 1992 Jun;34(11):1169-82 Underreaction to AIDS in Sub-Saharan Africa. Caldwell JC, Orubuloye IO, Caldwell P. Health Transition Centre, NCEPH, Australian National University, Canberra. In those parts of Sub-Saharan Africa most affected by the HIV/AIDS epidemic both public and private reaction to the seriousness of the epidemic have been less than might have been anticipated. This limited reaction weakens national, community and family responses to the epidemic and also reduces the pressure on international donors to provide adequate support. The paper first examines the reasons for underreaction by governments. These reasons include an assessment that successes will not be easily achieved, a reluctance to give leadership in areas of private sensitivity, an awareness of the fragility of the data base, a persistent feeling that it is a disease of foreign origin with a foreign overreaction to the situation in Africa, and the nature of the disease itself with a long latency period, obscure symptoms and an urban bias.

Soc Sci Med 1993
Dec;37(11):1401-13 AIDS action-research with women in Kinshasa, Zaire. Schoepf BG. AIDS has assumed epidemic proportions in Central Africa. Knowledge of culturally constructed gender relations and sexual meanings is crucial to developing prevention strategies and reducing the impact of AIDS. CONNAISSIDA, a transdisciplinary medical anthropology research project, developed culturally appropriate community-based empowerment workshops. These used cognitive, emotional and social stimulants to provoke critical reflection and action. Collaborative relationships developed in workshops were used to study sexual relations in many contexts. Significant changes in knowledge and action were observed. Nevertheless, economic necessity and inequality limited the ability of many women to avoid sexual risk. Economic crisis, structural adjustment and debt reimbursement policies have exacerbated poverty, particularly among women. Linking macrolevel political economy to microlevel sociocultural analysis shows how strategies adopted for survival contribute to sexual risk.

Soc Sci Med 1993 Feb;36(3):175-94 The competing discourses of HIV/AIDS in sub-Saharan Africa: discourses of rights and empowerment vs discourses of control and exclusion. Seidel G. University of Bradford, West Yorkshire, U.K. The competing discourses of HIV/AIDS circulating in sub-Saharan Africa are identified. These are medical, medico-moral, developmental (distinguishing between 'women in development' and gender and development perspectives), legal, ethical, and the rights discourse of groups living with HIV/AIDS and of African pressure groups. The analytical framework is that of discourse analysis as exemplified by Michel Foucault. The medical and medico-moral are identified as dominant. They shape the perceptions of the pandemic, our responses to it, and to those living with HIV/AIDS.

Soc Sci Med 1996 May;42(9):1283-96 Social vs biological: theories on the transmission of AIDS in Africa. Hunt CW. Department of Sociology, University of Utah, Salt Lake City 84112, USA. The present article critically examines these biological and social theories. It argues that the biological theories lack scientific support, lack sufficient evidential support, have an inequality of cause and effect, and fail to integrate the micro/macro. This article argues that the social theories also have some major difficulties including, in some cases, a failure to integrate the micro/macro and a lack of adequate or sufficient causation to produce the massive epidemic of AIDS in Africa. There are difficulties with the quality of evidence and support for the social theories and more research needs to be conducted, particularly in the form of retrospective studies, to determine the validity of various social theories which attempt to explain the epidemiological patterns of the AIDS epidemic in Africa.

Soc Sci Med 1996 May;42(9):1325-33 Notes on the socio-economic and cultural factors influencing the transmission of HIV in Botswana. MacDonald DS. Department of Sociology, University of Botswana, Gaborone. Botswana currently has one of the highest recorded incidences of HIV infection in Africa although AIDS was only first publicly recognized in 1985. By this time other countries in the region such as Malawi, Zambia and Uganda were already showing signs of epidemic levels of HIV. The rapid transmission of HIV in Botswana has been due to three main factors; the position of women in society, particularly their lack of power in negotiating sexual relationships: cultural attitudes to fertility; and social migration patterns. These three factors along with other, arguably more minor, ones have been shaped and mediated within the specific context of Botswana's rapid socio-economic development and cultural milieu.

Soc Sci Med 2001
Dec;53(11):1397-411
Voluntary counseling and
testing for couples: a high-
leverage intervention for
HIV/AIDS prevention in sub-
Saharan Africa. Painter TM.
Centers for Disease Control and
Prevention, National Center for
HIV, STD and TB Prevention,
Division of HIV/AIDS
Prevention-Surveillance and
Epidemiology, Atlanta, GA
30333, USA. tcp2@cdc.gov
Most HIV infections in sub-
Saharan Africa occur during
heterosexual intercourse
between persons in couple
relationships. Women who are
infected by HIV seropositive
partners risk infecting their
infants in turn. Despite their
salience as social contexts for
sexual activity and HIV
infection, couple relationships
have not been given adequate
attention by social/behavioral
research in sub-Saharan Africa.
Increasingly studies point to the
value of voluntary HIV
counseling and testing (VCT) as
a HIV prevention tool. Studies
in Africa frequently report that
VCT is associated with reduced
risk behaviors and lower rates of
seroconversion among HIV
serodiscordant couples. Many of
these studies point out that VCT
has considerable potential for
HIV prevention among other
heterosexual couples, and
recommend that VCT for
couples be practiced more
widely in Africa.

Stud Fam Plann 1998
Jun;29(2):154-66 Sexual
activity and contraceptive use:
the components of the
decisionmaking process. Gage
AJ. USAID, G/PHN/POP/P&E,
Washington, DC 20523-3601,
USA. In light of the social
consequences of early
childbearing, unplanned
pregnancy, and the transmission
of AIDS, a great need exists to
understand how adolescents
make sexual and reproductive
decisions. Drawing primarily on
literature from sub-Saharan
Africa, this article focuses on
three behavioral outcomes:
nonmarital sexual activity,
contraceptive use, and condom
use. It explores adolescent's
perceptions of the costs and
benefits of engaging in these
behaviors, their assessment of
their susceptibility to the
potential consequences of their
actions, and the role of family,
peer, and dyadic factors in
shaping their reproductive
decisions.

Stud Fam Plann 1998
Jun;29(2):210-32 The health
consequences of adolescent
sexual and fertility behavior in

sub-Saharan Africa. Zabin LS, Kiragu K. Department of Population Dynamics, Johns Hopkins School of Hygiene and Public Health, Baltimore, MD 21205, USA. This article reviews the literature on health consequences of adolescent sexual behavior and child-bearing in sub-Saharan Africa, and the social and cultural context in which they occur. It suggests that, in addressing the most serious health sequelae, sexual intercourse that occurs in early marriage and premaritally must both be considered. Some limitations of the data are noted.

Subst Use Misuse 1999 Feb;34(3):443-54 A review of literature on drug use in Sub-Saharan Africa countries and its economic and social implications. Affinnih YH. John Jay College of Criminal Justice, The City University of New York, New York 10019, USA. The drug problem in Africa cannot be seen as an isolated phenomenon but rather as part of the larger narcoscape which partakes of the fluid yet disjunctive qualities of Appadurai's landscapes. In this volatile environment, the transformation of Sub-Saharan Africa (SSA) nations from transit points in an international drug network to consumer countries seems inevitable. At the same time, Africa has undergone rapid economic and social changes that have facilitate this shift. A review of the literature reveals that there is a pressing need to investigate current trends and patterns of drug use in the countries of SSA.

Trans R Soc Trop Med Hyg 1993 Apr;87 Suppl 1:S19-22 No reason for complacency about the potential demographic impact of AIDS in Africa. Garnett GP, Anderson RM. Parasite Epidemiology Research Group, Imperial College, London, UK. Much uncertainty surrounds the likely demographic impact of AIDS in the worst afflicted regions of the developing world such as sub-Saharan Africa. Various research groups have published projections of future trends but these differ widely with respect to potential impact on net population growth rates. Pessimistic forecasts suggest that AIDS may reverse the sign of a 3% to 4% population growth rate before the establishment of HIV, over time periods of a few to many decades. Optimistic forecasts suggest a decline in population growth rates, but predict that a 3% growth rate before AIDS may be reduced by only about 50% over a period of a few decades. This paper reports new analyses of the demographic impact of AIDS, based on observed age-stratified prevalences of HIV-1 infection amongst women of child bearing age. It is assumed that the observed patterns reflect the final endemic state and the implications of this assumption for adult and infant mortality and female reproductive life expectancy are assessed. It is concluded that a variety of scenarios is possible, depending on the detail of assumptions concerning life expectancy before the arrival of AIDS, the incubation period of the disease, and the rate of vertical transmission.

Transfus Sci 1997 Jun;18(2):167-79 HIV and blood transfusion in sub-Saharan Africa. Fleming AF. University Teaching Hospital, Lusaka, Zambia. Blood transfusion services were poorly developed until the mid 1980s in most of sub-Saharan Africa, and were unable to provide adequate supplies of blood with acceptable safety. The pandemic of HIV was recognized seroepidemiologically from 1985 onwards. Blood transfusion was contributing from 10 to 15% to transmission in Africa. Groups at highest risk are children with malaria and anaemia, women with pregnancy-related haemorrhage or anaemia, victims of trauma and subjects with sickle-cell disease. Haemophiliacs are not a major risk group in comparison. Blood transfusion services have undoubtedly benefitted from the international, national and regional responses to the AIDS epidemic. Organizational structures have been established.

Transplantation 1997 Sep 15;64(5):669-73 Kaposi's sarcoma in transplant recipients. Penn I. University of Cincinnati Medical Center, Veterans Administration Medical Center, Ohio 45267, USA.

Trends Microbiol 1995 Jun;3(6):217-22 The epidemiology of HIV infection and AIDS in Africa. Van de Perre P. Laboratory of Retrovirology, Muraz Center, Bobo-Dioulasso, Burkina Faso. Only 10 years after it was first recognized in Africa, HIV infection is already the leading cause of adult death in many cities of the continent and has increased childhood mortality. This article reviews critical aspects of the dynamics of this epidemic, including routes of transmission, factors influencing the rate of transmission and strategies to combat this disaster.

Trop Doct 1998 Oct;28(4):243-5 Tuberculosis control in the face of the HIV epidemic. Harries AD, Nyirenda T, Banerjee A, Salaniponi FM, Boeree MJ. Programme Management Group, National Tuberculosis Control Programme, Lilongwe, Malawi.

Trop Geogr Med 1994;46(5):271-4 Tuberculosis in Africa--any news? van der Werf TS. Department of Pulmonary Diseases, University Hospital Groningen, The Netherlands. The tuberculosis situation in Africa in the AIDS era has become bleak. The tuberculosis incidence has increased in most sub-Saharan African countries, diagnosis has become more difficult, response to treatment, though initially good, is eventually less effective, and patient compliance, which has been a major problem in tuberculosis control before the HIV epidemic, has now become even more difficult. BCG vaccination, already ineffective before the AIDS era in preventing tuberculosis transmission, is now even less an appropriate tool in

tuberculosis control.

Trop Geogr Med 1995;47(2):78-81 Improving the quality of care for persons with HIV infection in sub-Saharan Africa. Colebunders R, Decock R, Mbeba MJ. Department of Microbiology, Institute of Tropical Medicine, Antwerp, Belgium. Caring for persons with HIV infection is particularly difficult in resource-poor countries. In order to improve the quality of care we first have to evaluate how such care is presently organized. We need a better assessment of the needs and demands of persons with HIV infection as well as their families. Care for persons with HIV/AIDS should be decentralized and home-based care in a non-stigmatizing way should be promoted. The fight against discrimination of persons with HIV should be intensified.

Trop Med Int Health 1996 Jun;1(3):295-304 HIV and India: looking into the abyss. Pais P. Department of Medicine, St John's Medical College Hospital, Bangalore, India. Serosurveillance of high risk groups started in India in October 1985. The first positive cases were detected in 1986. As of mid-1994, official figures stood at 15000 HIV positive cases and 559 cases of AIDS. This is most certainly an underestimate because of under reporting. Among high risk groups, prevalence has risen rapidly. Between 1986 and 1994, prevalence has risen from 1.6 to 40.0% in sex workers, 1.4 to 40% in STD clinics and 0 to 70% in i.v. drug abusers in various studies. The penetration into the general population is uncertain. As in Africa, infection has been mainly by heterosexual intercourse, with commercial sex workers, long distance truck drivers and migrant labour serving as vehicles of spread. Other routes of infection are transfusion of blood and blood products and i.v. drug use. Dependence on professional blood donors is the main cause of infected blood supplies. Ninety per cent of cases with HIV infection are aged between 15 and 45 years and belong to socioeconomically disadvantaged groups. The male to female ratio is 5:1, with female cases being mainly sex workers. The predominant virus is HIV-1 but cases with HIV-2 and mixed infection are being reported from port cities. The present situation in India is similar to the early pattern in Africa where a sharp increase in seroprevalence among high risk groups was followed by spread to the general population. Clinical AIDS is still infrequent.

Trop Med Int Health 1997 Feb;2(2):136-9 AIDS and hospital bed occupancy: an overview. Buve A. STD/HIV Research and Intervention Unit, Prins Leopold Institute of Tropical Medicine, Antwerpen, Belgium. In several countries of sub-Saharan Africa more than 10% of the adult population are infected with HIV, while in large towns such as Kampala, Lusaka, Blantyre, Kigali and Harare this proportion exceeds 25%. One of the most obvious consequences is the increased occupancy of hospital beds by patients with HIV infection, perhaps to the exclusion of patients with other ailments. This paper gives an overview of several hospital occupancy studies.

Trop Med Int Health 2000 Feb;5(2):85-7 Aggressive Kaposi's sarcoma in a 6-month-old African infant: case report and review of the literature. Manji KP, Amir H, Maduhu IZ. Department of Paediatrics, Muhimbili University College of Health Sciences, Dar-es-Salaam, Tanzania. kmanji@muchs.ac.tz Kaposi's sarcoma (KS), known to exist in Africa for a century now, was rare in children and unknown in the newborn. With the onset of the HIV/AIDS epidemic, a more aggressive, disseminated type of KS (AKS) was recognized. Recently KS was diagnosed in a 6-month-old infant in Tanzania. Data support the notion that HHSV8 infectivity can be potentiated with HIV infection and thus produce multiple lesions in different anatomical sites early in life. Furthermore, the available evidence would suggest a nonsexual route of HHSV8 infection, possibly from mother to fetus.

Trop Med Int Health 2000 Jul;5(7):A3-9 The global epidemiology of HIV/AIDS. Cock KM, Weiss HA. Division of HIV/AIDS Prevention, Surveillance and Epidemiology, Centers for Disease Control and Prevention, Atlanta, USA. The HIV pandemic continues to evolve, in both magnitude and diversity. In this paper, we briefly review the global epidemiology of HIV/AIDS, reflecting on the differences by region, and the challenges posed by the evolving epidemics in terms of prevention and surveillance. Despite the reduction in numbers of new AIDS cases in the US and Western Europe due to advances in treatment, a constant number of new HIV infections persists every year, with evidence that in some settings high-risk behaviour has increased, indicating failure in primary prevention.

Trop Med Parasitol 1995 Jun;46(2):69-71 Use of BCG in high prevalence areas for HIV. Felten MK, Leichsenring M. Tuberculosis Unit, University of Heidelberg Medical School, Germany. Recommendations state that, where the risk of tuberculosis is high, BCG should be administered to infants as early in life as possible, even if the mother is known to be HIV-infected. BCG should be withheld from individuals with symptomatic HIV infections.

Ugeskr Laeger 1995 Sep 18;157(38):5232-6 Kaposi sarcoma. An epidemiological perspective [Article in Danish] Lecker S, Melbye M. Center for epidemiologisk grundforskning, Statens Seruminstitut, Kobenhavn. Prior to the 1980s, Kaposi's sarcoma was a rare tumour diagnosed three to four times more frequently among men than women. It was primarily seen among elderly men of Mediterranean or Jewish descent, in well-defined areas of Central Africa, or more scattered as individual cases with underlying immunosuppression. Geographical restrictions and suggested associations with certain HLA-types gave rise to early speculations of a genetic component involved in its etiology. With the AIDS epidemic, the epidemiology of Kaposi's sarcoma changed drastically. Although diagnosed among AIDS patients that are transfusion recipients, intravenous drug users and haemophiliacs, Kaposi's sarcoma is primarily found in homosexual men with AIDS among whom the risk has increased to 100,000 compared to the general population. Specific behaviours linked to homosexual men have been sought to explain this relationship, but accumulating evidence favours the involvement of an infectious agent in the etiology of Kaposi's sarcoma.

Ugeskr Laeger 1996 Mar 18;158(12):1662-6 Infection with human immunodeficiency virus type 2--HIV-2 [Article in Danish] Christiansen CB. Virologisk afdeling, Statens Seruminstitut, Kobenhavn. The majority of patients with HIV-2

infection come from West Africa or have had sexual contact with a person from there, as HIV-2 is prevalent in this area. HIV-2 is phylogenetically closer related to SIVsm and SIVmac than to HIV-1. HIV-2 is mainly transmitted by heterosexual contact, whereas the risk of mother-to-child infection is very low. Nine cases of HIV-2 infection have been diagnosed in Denmark. Out of these, seven are from West Africa and two have been infected in Denmark by individuals from West Africa.

Ugeskr Laeger 1997 Feb 24;159(9):1233-8 Tuberculosis and the HIV pandemic. Risk of nosocomial tuberculosis infection [Article in Danish] Pedersen C, Kolmos HJ, Nielsen JO. Klinisk mikrobiologisk afdeling, Hvidovre Hospital. Spread of human immunodeficiency virus (HIV) infection has had a major impact on the epidemiology of tuberculosis. In several African countries the incidence of tuberculosis has doubled, and the prevalence of HIV infection among patients with tuberculosis is 20 to 60%. A similar change has occurred in some developed countries. Several factors, including HIV infection, have contributed to this change. Tuberculosis among HIV infected patients is probably more often a result of a new infection with Mycobacterium tuberculosis than reactivation of a latent infection.

Ugeskr Laeger 2000 Nov 13;162(46):6203-7 Leishmaniasis [Article in Danish] Kemp M, Theander TG. Klinisk mikrobiologisk afdeling, H:S Hvidovre Hospital. MKE@dadlnet.dk Leishmania parasites are obligate intracellular protozoa, that produce clinical pictures, ranging from localised, self-healing ulcers to systemic, lethal diseases. The diseases caused by the parasites can be divided into cutaneous, mucocutaneous, and visceral leishmaniasis. Recovery from the infection often leaves lifelong immunity. Leishmaniasis may occur in individuals who have been to the Mediterranean countries, the countries on the Horn of Africa, the Arabian Peninsula, parts of Asia, and South and Central America. Co-infection of Leishmania parasites and HIV is a special problem. Leishmaniasis can be treated with pentavalent compounds of antimony, but other drugs, including amphotericin B, are also affective.

Vaccine 2001 Mar 21;19(17-19):2210-5 Current progress in the development of human immunodeficiency virus vaccines: research and clinical trials. Klein M. Aventis Pasteur, Campus Merieux, 1541 Avenue Marcel Merieux, 69280, Marcy l'Etoile, France. Michel.Klein@aventis.com In spite of extensive prevention programs, the HIV pandemic is still spreading worldwide, particularly in developing countries. AIDS is the leading cause of death in Africa and the fourth cause worldwide. WHO estimates that there are 16000 new cases of HIV infection daily and that 100 million individuals will be infected during the next decade. In spite of the spectacular results of triple therapy, the best strategy for controlling the HIV epidemics remains the development of an efficacious prophylactic vaccine.

Wien Klin Wochenschr 1995;107(3):85-90 Transmission of HIV infection [Article in German] Tomaso H, Reisinger EC, Grasmug E, Ramschak H, Krejs GJ. Medizinische Universitatsklinik der Karl-Franzens-Universitat, Graz. The increasing number of human immuno-deficiency virus (HIV) infections and the shift from traditional risk groups to the general population give reason for reviewing the routes and risks of virus transmission. In Africa HIV is transmitted mainly by heterosexual contact; in Europe and the USA homosexuality is still the leading cause of infection, however, heterosexual transmission is increasing dramatically. The heterogeneity of HIV strains and host factors may contribute to the progression of HIF infection to AIDS.

Zentralbl Bakteriol 1995 Nov;283(1):5-13 On the development of mycobacterial infections. I. A review concerning the common situation. Schutt-Gerowitt H. Institut fur Medizinische Mikrobiologie und Hygiene, Universitat zu Koln, Germany. In this review concerning the common situation of mycobacterial infections the following problems are discussed: (1) The worldwide epidemiological situation of tuberculosis reveals an increase in the developing countries but even in some industrialized countries like the United States. The reasons for this development are mainly socioeconomic factors. (2) The association between tuberculosis and HIV infection has caused in general a marked increase in the incidence of tuberculosis in some countries. Because of its ability to destroy the immune system, HIV is a significant risk factor for the progression of tuberculosis infection as a clinical disease. Taking into account that 5 million persons worldwide are infected with tuberculosis as well as with HIV (most of them living in the Sub-Saharan Africa), enormous future problems can be anticipated. (3) The new fear of tuberculosis has resulted mainly from reports about outbreaks with multidrug resistant strains of Mycobacterium tuberculosis in the United States. These strains are at least resistant to the most important antituberculotic drugs isoniacid and rifampicin. The frequency of multidrug-resistant tuberculosis in the USA is reported to be overall 3-7%, however for New York 19% is estimated. The main reason for this development is inadequate chemotherapy mostly due to poor compliance. Therefore in the United States the directly observed therapy has been established. Complete and reliable reports of the resistance situation in other countries are not available because most of these have no resistance surveillance programs. (4) As immunocompromised patients become more numerous, the importance of nontuberculous mycobacteria has significantly increased. Mainly organisms of the Mycobacterium avium-intracellulare complex play a special role as opportunistic pathogens for AIDS patients in later stages of their disease. Therapy for these infections is problematic due to the high resistance of most ubiquitous mycobacteria to antituberculotic drugs. (5) New laboratory techniques have shortened the detection time (radiometric culture systems) and the time needed for the identification of the most important mycobacteria species (DNA probes).

Zentralbl Hyg Umweltmed 1993 Feb;194(1-2):152-61
Persistence of mycobacteria in the host: epidemiology, immunopathology and prophylaxis [Article in German] Mauch H. Institut fur Mikrobiologie, Immunologie und Laboratoriumsmedizin, Krankenhaus Zehlendorf-Heckeshorn, Berlin.

Tuberculosis continues to be one of the major causes of morbidity and mortality in the developed and developing countries. There are more than 5000 cases of active open tuberculous lung disease in Germany. Worldwide approximately 10 million persons get tuberculous infections each year. Other not yet infected people in the community are endangered by this disease, especially those with immunodeficiency e.g. AIDS-patients or tumor patients. M. tuberculosis with its unique glycolipid cell wall is fairly resistant against the immune system. Only specialized activated macrophages are able to inhibit its growth. The bacteris may persist for years in the living body, probably in granulomas. A positive tuberculin-reaction indicates an infection and persistance of mycobacteria but does not prove a disease.

Zhonghua Liu Xing Bing Xue Za Zhi 1997 Apr;18(2):102-5
Study of the reasons for spread of communicable diseases [Article in Chinese] Wei CY.

AUTHOR INDEX

C

I

H

J

S

TITLE INDEX

B

R

S

W

U

V

SUBJECT INDEX

B

C

E

F

G

Q

R

T

U

V

W

Y

Z